Hereditary Hemorrhagic Telangiectasia: Diagnosis and Management

Hereditary Hemorrhagic Telangiectasia: Diagnosis and Management

Editor

Angel M. Cuesta

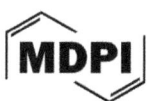

Basel • Beijing • Wuhan • Barcelona • Belgrade • Novi Sad • Cluj • Manchester

Editor
Angel M. Cuesta
Complutense University of Madrid
Madrid
Spain

Editorial Office
MDPI
St. Alban-Anlage 66
4052 Basel, Switzerland

This is a reprint of articles from the Special Issue published online in the open access journal *Journal of Clinical Medicine* (ISSN 2077-0383) (available at: https://www.mdpi.com/journal/jcm/special_issues/H_H_T).

For citation purposes, cite each article independently as indicated on the article page online and as indicated below:

Lastname, A.A.; Lastname, B.B. Article Title. *Journal Name* **Year**, *Volume Number*, Page Range.

ISBN 978-3-0365-9901-4 (Hbk)
ISBN 978-3-0365-9902-1 (PDF)
doi.org/10.3390/books978-3-0365-9902-1

© 2024 by the authors. Articles in this book are Open Access and distributed under the Creative Commons Attribution (CC BY) license. The book as a whole is distributed by MDPI under the terms and conditions of the Creative Commons Attribution-NonCommercial-NoDerivs (CC BY-NC-ND) license.

Contents

About the Editor vii

Angel M. Cuesta
Hereditary Hemorrhagic Telangiectasia: Diagnosis and Management
Reprinted from: *J. Clin. Med.* **2022**, *11*, 4698, doi:10.3390/jcm11164698 1

**Suriel Errasti Díaz, Mercedes Peñalva, Lucía Recio-Poveda, Susana Vilches,
Juan Casado-Vela, Julián Pérez Pérez, et al.**
A Novel Splicing Mutation in the *ACVRL1/ALK1* Gene as a Cause of HHT2
Reprinted from: *J. Clin. Med.* **2022**, *11*, 3035, doi:10.3390/jcm11113053 4

Eleonora Gaetani, Elisabetta Peppucci, Fabiana Agostini, Luigi Di Martino, Emanuela Lucci Cordisco, Carmelo L. Sturiale, et al.
Distribution of Cerebrovascular Phenotypes According to Variants of the *ENG* and *ACVRL1* Genes in Subjects with Hereditary Hemorrhagic Telangiectasia
Reprinted from: *J. Clin. Med.* **2022**, *11*, 2685, doi:10.3390/jcm11102685 14

**Kornelia E. C. Andorfer, Caroline T. Seebauer, Carolin Dienemann, Steven C. Marcrum,
René Fischer, Christopher Bohr and Thomas S. Kühnel**
HHT-Related Epistaxis and Pregnancy—A Retrospective Survey and Recommendations for Management from an Otorhinolaryngology Perspective
Reprinted from: *J. Clin. Med.* **2022**, *11*, 2178, doi:10.3390/jcm11082178 22

**Caroline T. Seebauer, Viola Freigang, Franziska E. Schwan, René Fischer, Christopher Bohr,
Thomas S. Kühnel and Kornelia E. C. Andorfer**
Hereditary Hemorrhagic Telangiectasia: Success of the Osler Calendar for Documentation of Treatment and Course of Disease
Reprinted from: *J. Clin. Med.* **2021**, *10*, 4720, doi:10.3390/jcm10204720 35

**Sol Marcos, Luisa María Botella, Virginia Albiñana, Agustina Arbia and
Anna María de Rosales**
Sclerotherapy on Demand with Polidocanol to Treat HHT Nosebleeds
Reprinted from: *J. Clin. Med.* **2021**, *10*, 3845, doi:10.3390/jcm10173845 46

**Tamás Major, Zsuzsanna Bereczky, Réka Gindele, Gábor Balogh, Benedek Rácz,
László Bora, et al.**
Current Status of Clinical and Genetic Screening of Hereditary Hemorrhagic Telangiectasia Families in Hungary
Reprinted from: *J. Clin. Med.* **2021**, *10*, 3774, doi:10.3390/jcm10173774 57

Eleonora Gaetani, Fabiana Agostini, Luigi Di Martino, Denis Occhipinti, Giulio Cesare Passali, Mariaconsiglia Santantonio, et al.
Beneficial Effects of Remote Medical Care for Patients with Hereditary Hemorrhagic Telangiectasia during the COVID-19 Pandemic
Reprinted from: *J. Clin. Med.* **2021**, *10*, 2311, doi:10.3390/jcm10112311 74

**Freya Droege, Andreas Stang, Kruthika Thangavelu, Carolin Lueb, Stephan Lang,
Michael Xydakis and Urban Geisthoff**
Restless Leg Syndrome Is Underdiagnosed in Hereditary Hemorrhagic Telangiectasia—Results of an Online Survey
Reprinted from: *J. Clin. Med.* **2021**, *10*, 1993, doi:10.3390/jcm10091993 81

Sol Marcos, Virginia Albiñana, Lucia Recio-Poveda, Belisa Tarazona, María Patrocinio Verde-González, et al.
SARS-CoV-2 Infection in Hereditary Hemorrhagic Telangiectasia Patients Suggests Less Clinical Impact Than in the General Population
Reprinted from: *J. Clin. Med.* **2021**, *10*, 1884, doi:10.3390/jcm10091884 . . . . **90**

Tamás Major, Réka Gindele, Gábor Balogh, Péter Bárdossy and Zsuzsanna Bereczky
Founder Effects in Hereditary Hemorrhagic Telangiectasia
Reprinted from: *J. Clin. Med.* **2021**, *10*, 1682, doi:10.3390/jcm10081682 . . . . **103**

About the Editor

Angel M. Cuesta

Graduated on Life Sciences (Biochemistry and Molecular Biology) in 2003, he initiated his PhD studies at University Hospital Puerta de Hierro working of recombinant multivalent and multispecific antibodies.

In 2009 he obtained his PhD degree and in 2011 he moved to the Buchman Institute for Molecular Life Sciences (Excellence Cluster Frankfurt Goethe-Univ) in Germany. There, he established, managed, and developed an In Vivo Cancer Imaging facility for new cancer animal models; focused on glioblastoma (GBM) and lung carcinoma.

On 2017, he combined a research position at the Centro de Investigaciones Biológicas Margarita Salas-CSIC with teaching activities as Associate Lecturer at the Universidad Complutense de Madrid (UCM). Along this time, he developed translational research on two rare diseases von Hippel-Lindau (VHL) and Hereditary hemorrhagic telangiectasia (HHT).

Recently, in 2023 he got a permanent position as Assistant Professor at UCM. There he continues working on VHL, HHT and Glioblastoma, another rare cancer. Moreover, he also works on unravelling the role of C3G in GBM and liver diseases.

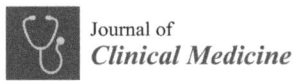

Editorial
Hereditary Hemorrhagic Telangiectasia: Diagnosis and Management

Angel M. Cuesta [1,2]

1 Departamento de Bioquímica y Biología Molecular, Facultad de Farmacia, Complutense University of Madrid, 28040 Madrid, Spain; angcuest@ucm.es
2 CIBERER, Centro de Investigación Biomédica en Red de Enfermedades Raras, Unidad 707, Instituto de Salud Carlos III (ISCIII), 28029 Madrid, Spain

Hereditary hemorrhagic telangiectasia (HHT), or Rendu-Osler-Weber syndrome, is a dominantly inheritable rare disease with a prevalence of 1:5000–10,000 inhabitants.

The diagnosis of HHT follows the Curaçao diagnostic criteria [1]:
1. NOSEBLEEDS (epistaxis) that are spontaneous and recurrent.
2. (Multiple) TELANGIECTASES at characteristic sites, including the lips, oral cavity, fingers and nose.
3. INTERNAL LESIONS: arteriovenous malformations (AVMs) or telangiectases in the stomach, lungs, liver, brain and spinal cord.
4. FAMILY HISTORY: a first-degree relative with HHT according to these criteria.

When the patient meets at least three of these criteria, he/she is considered to have definitive HHT.

To date, three subtypes of HHT have been described. HHT type 1 refers to mutations of the endoglin gene *ENG*; HHT type 2 refers to mutations of the activin A receptor, similar to the type-1 *ACVRL1* gene; and the third type, known as juvenile polyposis–hereditary hemorrhagic telangiectasia (JPHT or JPHHT) overlap syndrome, refers to mutations of the gene *MADH 4*. There are two other subtypes (HHT-3 and HHT-4) whose mutations have not yet been completely identified, but it is known that they are located in the 5q31.3–q32 and 7p14 chromosomal regions, respectively [2,3].

This Special Issue (SI), with nine original articles and one review, focuses on "Diagnosis and Management." Management is not possible without a correct diagnosis. However, this obvious statement ignores the fact that the average time taken for a diagnosis of HHT to be established is 27 years, as noted by Major, T. et al., with the average diagnosis in Hungary being obtained over periods between 22.6 and 29.1 years [4].

This phenomenon occurs in developed countries, but we cannot forget that we still need to address the terra incognita. We cannot forget about developing or emerging countries, where the prevalence should be similar, and the founder effects may be reinforced by physical boundaries [5], but the medical assistance is far from the desired level.

In this sense, the international collaboration reported by Errasti Díaz et al. highlights the difficulties of performing a rather easy genetic test for a new mutation HHT in Peru [6]. In addition to the novelty of this new mutation, it should also shed light on and inspire international collaboration, due to the fact that the number of inhabitants can lead to thousands of HHT patients (and patients with many other rare diseases) remaining unidentified.

Major, T. et al. assert that society is lacking in knowledge of HHT disease and that this is related to the unawareness of HHT within the medical community [4]. I would only add that, as seen in this SI, those physicians who are aware of rare diseases such as HHT they never let their patients down and always do their best to help them.

Gaetani E. et al. describe a very interesting genotype–phenotype correlation between cerebrovascular malformations in HHT patients. This kind of study could help to eliminate the differences identified in 2020 regarding the recommendations for screening children for brain VMs [7,8].

Citation: Cuesta, A.M. Hereditary Hemorrhagic Telangiectasia: Diagnosis and Management. *J. Clin. Med.* **2022**, *11*, 4698. https://doi.org/10.3390/jcm11164698

Received: 1 August 2022
Accepted: 8 August 2022
Published: 11 August 2022

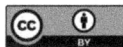

Copyright: © 2022 by the author. Licensee MDPI, Basel, Switzerland. This article is an open access article distributed under the terms and conditions of the Creative Commons Attribution (CC BY) license (https://creativecommons.org/licenses/by/4.0/).

Andorfer et al. present a retrospective study on the evolution and management of HHT disease in pregnant HHT patients, indicating that, even that the risks are low, better procedures should be implemented to minimize the negative effects of the disorder [9].

COVID-19, as is the case worldwide, has also affected HHT patients. In this SI, one can read about an interesting Spanish study, in which HHT patients appeared to be less affected by the viral infection due to a minor cytokine storm [10]. It would be incredibly useful if a larger and international retrospective study were to confirm these data, which were obtained from 138 HHT patients. Moreover, the results of an Italian observational study on the remote care of HHT patients identified the benefits and rapid response of this kind of assistance [11].

Lastly, but not least, this SI reports on different aspects of the management of HHT patients aiming to improve their quality of life. In Germany, Seebauer et al. studied the benefits of using an HHT disease calendar, indicating the improvement of the cross-communication between patients and clinicians, but also highlighting the lack of knowledge about the disease among the patients, as indicated previously in [12]. Droege et al. described the underestimation of restless leg syndrome in HHT patients as a consequence of recurrent epistaxis and internal bleedings and highlighted the need for a treatment [13].

Moreover, the management of this disease for a better quality of life of the patients involves the improvement or the creation of simple, rapid and cheap treatments. In this sense, Marcos et al. demonstrated the benefits of sclerotherapy on demand, as observed in 105 patients [14].

Finally, we can conclude that this SI covers key areas of the disease that must be solved in the near future, such as the need for international collaboration, the management of cerebrovascular malformations, and the improvement of the daily life of the patients through educational programs on the disease, remote care and specialized on-demand assistance.

We hope that our readers enjoy this SI, which was revised by international experts in the basic research and clinics of HHT disease.

Funding: This research received no external funding.

Conflicts of Interest: The author declare no conflict of interest.

References

1. Shovlin, C.L.; Guttmacher, A.E.; Buscarini, E.; Faughnan, M.E.; Hyland, R.H.; Westermann, C.J.; Kjeldsen, A.D.; Plauchu, H. Diagnostic criteria for hereditary hemorrhagic telangiectasia (Rendu-Osler-Weber syndrome). *Am. J. Med. Genet.* **2000**, *91*, 66–67. [CrossRef]
2. Cole, S.G.; Begbie, M.E.; Wallace, G.M.F.; Shovlin, C.L. A new locus for hereditary haemorrhagic telangiectasia (HHT3) maps to chromosome 5. *J. Med. Genet.* **2005**, *42*, 577–582. [CrossRef] [PubMed]
3. Bayrak-Toydemir, P.; McDonald, J.; Akarsu, N.; Toydemir, R.M.; Calderon, F.; Tuncali, T.; Tang, W.; Miller, F.; Mao, R. A fourth locus for hereditary hemorrhagic telangiectasia maps to chromosome 7. *Am. J. Med. Genet. Part A* **2006**, *140*, 2155–2162. [CrossRef] [PubMed]
4. Major, T.; Bereczky, Z.; Gindele, R.; Balogh, G.; Rácz, B.; Bora, L.; Kézsmárki, Z.; Brúgós, B.; Pfliegler, G. Current Status of Clinical and Genetic Screening of Hereditary Hemorrhagic Telangiectasia Families in Hungary. *J. Clin. Med.* **2021**, *10*, 3774. [CrossRef] [PubMed]
5. Major, T.; Gindele, R.; Balogh, G.; Bárdossy, P.; Bereczky, Z. Founder Effects in Hereditary Hemorrhagic Telangiectasia. *J. Clin. Med.* **2021**, *10*, 1682. [CrossRef] [PubMed]
6. Errasti Díaz, S.; Peñalva, M.; Recio-Poveda, L.; Vilches, S.; Casado-Vela, J.; Pérez Pérez, J.; Botella, L.M.; Albiñana, V.; Cuesta, A.M. A Novel Splicing Mutation in the ACVRL1/ALK1 Gene as a Cause of HHT2. *J. Clin. Med.* **2022**, *11*, 3053. [CrossRef] [PubMed]
7. Gaetani, E.; Peppucci, E.; Agostini, F.; Di Martino, L.; Cordisco, E.L.; Sturiale, C.L.; Puca, A.; Porfidia, A.; Alexandre, A.; Pedicelli, A.; et al. Distribution of Cerebrovascular Phenotypes According to Variants of the *ENG* and *ACVRL1* Genes in Subjects with Hereditary Hemorrhagic Telangiectasia. *J. Clin. Med.* **2022**, *11*, 2685. [CrossRef] [PubMed]
8. Faughnan, M.E.; Mager, J.J.; Hetts, S.W.; Palda, V.A.; Lang-Robertson, K.; Buscarini, E.; Deslandres, E.; Kasthuri, R.S.; Lausman, A.; Poetker, D.; et al. Second International Guidelines for the Diagnosis and Management of Hereditary Hemorrhagic Telangiectasia. *Ann. Intern. Med.* **2020**, *173*, 989–1001. [CrossRef]
9. Andorfer, K.E.C.; Seebauer, C.T.; Dienemann, C.; Marcrum, S.C.; Fischer, R.; Bohr, C.; Kühnel, T.S. HHT-Related Epistaxis and Pregnancy—A Retrospective Survey and Recommendations for Management from an Otorhinolaryngology Perspective. *J. Clin. Med.* **2022**, *11*, 2178. [CrossRef] [PubMed]

10. Marcos, S.; Albiñana, V.; Recio-Poveda, L.; Tarazona, B.; Verde-González, M.P.; Ojeda-Fernández, L.; Botella, L.M. SARS-CoV-2 Infection in Hereditary Hemorrhagic Telangiectasia Patients Suggests Less Clinical Impact than in the General Population. *J. Clin. Med.* **2021**, *10*, 1884. [CrossRef] [PubMed]
11. Gaetani, E.; Agostini, F.; Di Martino, L.; Occhipinti, D.; Passali, G.; Santantonio, M.; Marano, G.; Mazza, M.; Pola, R.; on behalf of the Multidisciplinary Gemelli Group for HHT. Beneficial Effects of Remote Medical Care for Patients with Hereditary Hemorrhagic Telangiectasia during the COVID-19 Pandemic. *J. Clin. Med.* **2021**, *10*, 2311. [CrossRef] [PubMed]
12. Seebauer, C.T.; Freigang, V.; Schwan, F.E.; Fischer, R.; Bohr, C.; Kühnel, T.S.; Andorfer, K.E.C. Hereditary Hemorrhagic Telangiectasia: Success of the Osler Calendar for Documentation of Treatment and Course of Disease. *J. Clin. Med.* **2021**, *10*, 4720. [CrossRef] [PubMed]
13. Droege, F.; Stang, A.; Thangavelu, K.; Lueb, C.; Lang, S.; Xydakis, M.; Geisthoff, U. Restless Leg Syndrome Is Underdiagnosed in Hereditary Hemorrhagic Telangiectasia—Results of an Online Survey. *J. Clin. Med.* **2021**, *10*, 1993. [CrossRef] [PubMed]
14. Marcos, S.; Botella, L.M.; Albiñana, V.; Arbia, A.; de Rosales, A.M. Sclerotherapy on Demand with Polidocanol to Treat HHT Nosebleeds. *J. Clin. Med.* **2021**, *10*, 3845. [CrossRef] [PubMed]

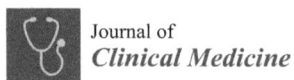

Article

A Novel Splicing Mutation in the *ACVRL1/ALK1* Gene as a Cause of HHT2

Suriel Errasti Díaz [1], Mercedes Peñalva [2], Lucía Recio-Poveda [2,3], Susana Vilches [4], Juan Casado-Vela [5,6], Julián Pérez Pérez [4], Luisa María Botella [2,3], Virginia Albiñana [2,3,*] and Angel M. Cuesta [3,7,*]

1. Departamento Hematología, Instituto Nacional de Enfermedades Neoplásicas, Lima 15038, Peru; suriel_ed@hotmail.com
2. Departamento Biomedicina Molecular, Centro de Investigaciones Biológicas Margarita Salas (CIB), Consejo Superior de Investigaciones Científicas (CSIC), 280406 Madrid, Spain; mpenalva@ucm.es (M.P.); luciarecio@hotmail.com (L.R.-P.); cibluisa@cib.csic.es (L.M.B.)
3. CIBERER, Unidad 707, Instituto de Salud Carlos III (ISCIII), 28029 Madrid, Spain
4. Laboratorio Diagnóstico Genético Secugen SL, CIB, CSIC, 28040 Madrid, Spain; s.vilches@secugen.es (S.V.); j.perez@secugen.es (J.P.P.)
5. Facultad de Ciencias Experimentales, Universidad Francisco de Vitoria, Pozuelo, 28223 Madrid, Spain; jucasado@ing.uc3m.es
6. Departamento Bioingeniería, Escuela Politécnica Superior, Universidad Carlos III de Madrid, 28911 Madrid, Spain
7. Departamento de Bioquímica y Biología Molecular, Facultad de Farmacia, Universidad Complutense de Madrid, 28040 Madrid, Spain
* Correspondence: vir_albi_di@yahoo.es (V.A.); angcuest@ucm.es (A.M.C.)

Abstract: Hereditary Hemorrhagic Telangiectasia (HHT) is a rare disorder of vascular development. Common manifestations include epistaxis, telangiectasias and arteriovenous malformations in multiple organs. Different deletions or nonsense mutations have been described in the ENG (HHT1) or ACVRL1/ALK1 (HHT2) genes, all affecting endothelial homeostasis. A novel mutation in *ACVRL1/ALK1* has been identified in a Peruvian family with a clinical history compatible to HHT. Subsequently, 23 DNA samples from oral exchanges (buccal swaps) of the immediate family members were analyzed together with their clinical histories. A routine cDNA PCR followed by comparative DNA sequencing between the founder and another healthy family member showed the presence of the aforementioned specific mutation. The single mutation detected (c.525 + 1G > T) affects the consensus splice junction immediately after exon 4, provokes anomalous splicing and leads to the inclusion of intron IV between exons 4 and 5 in the *ACVRL1/ALK1* mRNA and, therefore, to *ALK1* haploinsufficiency. Complete sequencing determined that 10 of the 25 family members analyzed were affected by the same mutation. Notably, the approach described in this report could be used as a diagnostic technique, easily incorporated in clinical practice in developing countries and easily extrapolated to other patients carrying such a mutation.

Keywords: *ACVRL1/ALK1*; hereditary hemorrhagic telangiectasia; splicing mutation; Osler-Weber-Rendu disease

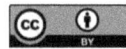

1. Introduction

Hereditary Hemorrhagic Telangiectasia (HHT), also known as Osler-Weber-Rendu disease, is an autosomal dominant multisystemic vascular dysplasia. Patients with HHT may present multiple symptoms, thus, interfering with efficient clinical diagnosis and optimal patient treatment. Diagnosis is made clinically using the Curaçao criteria: epistaxis (nosebleeds that increase in frequency and quantity with age and are the most common symptom), telangiectases (red-purple spots on the face, lips, mucosa, and fingers), visceral arteriovenous malformations (AVMs) in the lungs, brain, and liver, being the result of abnormal connections between arteries and veins, where the capillary bed has disappeared [1–3], and family history. The most severe symptoms include anemia, gastrointestinal bleeding, and complications due to AVMs [3,4]. Typically, if three of the four criteria are present, the patient is diagnosed with HHT [2,5].

Depending on the gene locus affected by mutation, different types of HHT have been reported. The most frequent subtypes, HHT1 and HHT2, are caused by mutations in the *Endoglin (ENG)* and *Activin Receptor-Like Kinase 1 (ACVRL1/ALK1)* genes, respectively, accounting for almost 90% of all HHT cases [6].

HHT3 and HHT4 have been mapped by linkage studies to chromosomal regions 5q31.3-q32 and 7p14, respectively, but no gene has been identified yet [7,8]. Mutations in the *GDF2* gene have been related to HHT-like disease [4,9]. Finally, another gene, *MADH4/SMAD4,* has been identified as being responsible for a combined syndrome, including HHT and juvenile polyposis [10].

A patient with HHT, hereafter the proband, diagnosed by his Health Care Provider in Lima (Peru), according to Curaçao criteria (mentioned above), came for epistaxis treatment to Madrid (Spain). Blood samples were taken from him and from an unaffected relative (with no apparent symptoms) for further genetic analysis. Strikingly, the genetic diagnosis of the HHT patient revealed the presence of a previously unreported mutation, c.525 + 1G > T, affecting the consensus splice site after exon 4 of the *ACVRL1/ALK1* gene. Subsequently, we decided to perform a genetic analysis on all the Peruvian family members who wanted to participate in the study (23 more individuals). For this purpose, buccal swaps were used to obtain the samples in Peru and they were sent to our lab.

In this work, we present the genetic diagnosis, the phenotypic manifestations, of the largest cohort of HHT published so far in Peru. We also demonstrate here, the anomalous presence of the intron IV of *ACVRL1* in the transcripts of the HHT sample, according to the prediction of abnormal splicing due to the mutation present in the family analyzed in this report. Finally, we believe that this is an example of collaboration in the diagnoses of rare diseases, such as HHT, with developing countries that should be emulated.

2. Materials and Methods

2.1. Human Samples

The entire procedure was approved by the ethical committee of the National Agency of Research in Spain (CSIC), with the reference 075/2017. Blood samples from members of a Peruvian family (a proband meeting HHT Curaçao criteria and a healthy relative) with HHT history were sent from the Hospital Universitario Fundación Alcorcón (HUFA) to our laboratory. Informed consent from both donors was obtained. In addition, 23 buccal swaps samples from direct relatives of the proband (index case) were sent from Peru to our laboratory, with the informed consent of each of the sample donors.

2.2. Peripheral Blood Mononuclear Cells (PBMCs) Extraction

A blood gradient was made from the patient's sample by adding 8 mL of blood on a bed of 4 mL of Ficoll. To achieve separation of the blood components, samples were centrifuged for 20 min at $1000\times$ g without brake. Next, the fraction containing the Peripheral Blood Mononuclear Cells (PBMC) was extracted and, together with 5 mL of Phosphate-Buffered Saline (PBS), centrifuged at 1500 rpm for 5 min. The supernatant was removed. The cell pellet was used for two purposes: DNA extraction and cell cultures.

2.3. DNA Total Extraction and Sequencing

Total DNA was extracted from Peripheral Blood Mononuclear Cells using the QIAamp Mini Kit (Qiagen, Germany) and following the manufacturer indications.

In the case of buccal swaps DNA extraction was carried out with the same kit, but the first step of lysis was performed with a greater volume as recommended, and lysis was prolonged for 12 h at 56 °C to ensure the highest recovery.

The obtained DNA was subjected to PCR amplification and Sanger sequencing in the case of index case for *ACVRL1/ALK1* and *ENG* exons and intron–exons boundaries, as described in Fernandez-L et al., 2006 [11]. Then, sequences were compared to reference sequences in the databank for *ACVRL1/ALK1* and *ENG*. In the case of direct relatives, exon 4 of *ACVRL1/ALK1* was subjected to PCR amplification using the HotMaster Taq DNA Polymerase (5 Prime, Germany) and subsequent Sanger capillary sequencing [12].

2.4. RNA Expression Analysis in Peripheral Blood Mononuclear Cells: RNA Extraction, Retrotranscription and qPCR

Cells isolated after Ficoll gradient centrifugation of 10 mL peripheral blood were plated in single wells of P-6 culture plates and cultured in 2 mL DMEM supplemented with 10% Fetal Bovine Serum (FBS).

After 48 h, adherent cells were detached and centrifuged at 1500 rpm for 5 min. Pellets were subjected to RNA extraction using the NucleoSpin RNA purification kit (Macherey-Nagel GmbH&Co., Düren, Germany), following the manufacturer protocol. Around 1 µg of RNA was retrotranscribed using the Applied Biosystems kit (Thermo Fisher Scientific, Waltham, MA, USA).

Quantitative PCR was performed by FastStart Essential DNA Green Master (Roche, Switzerland) to amplify *β-Actin* and *18S* RNA as housekeeping genes and *ENG* and *ACVRL1/ALK1* as test genes using the primers shown in the following Table 1. Samples were run in triplicate.

Table 1. Primers used for q-PCR assays.

Gene	Fwd 5′-3′	Rev 5′-3′
18S	CTAACACGGGAAACCTCAC	CGCTCCACCAACTAAGAACG
ACVRL1/ALK1	ATCTGAGCAGGGCGACAGC	GAGGGACACCACGTCAGT
ENG	AGCCTCAGCCCCACAAGT	GTCACCTCGTCCCTCTCG
β-actin	AGCCTCGCCTTTGCCGA	CTGGTGCCTGGGGCG

3. Results

3.1. Genetic Analysis of an HHT Family from Peru

The HHT proband was a 62-year-old Peruvian male, diagnosed with HHT by his clinician. The diagnosis fit the Curaçao criteria: nosebleeds, gastric bleeds (AVMs detected by endoscopy), anemia, and family history of nosebleeds. His main problem was anemia, requiring transfusions from time to time due to his severe epistaxis. The patient travelled from Peru to be treated of his epistaxis by sclerotherapy performed by an HHT-ENT referrer at the Hospital Universitario Fundación Alcorcón (HUFA) [13]. In addition, the proband was examined for the presence of AVMs in lung, brain, and liver. No AVMs were found in brain or lung and no hepatic arteriovenous malformations (HAVM) were found. At the same time, blood was extracted for genetic diagnosis. Routine sequencing started with the *ACVRL1/ALK1* gene, due to the absence of pulmonary arteriovenous malformations (PAVMs), which are rare in HHT2, but quite common in HHT1 [14]. Subsequently, *endoglin* was also sequenced in case a mutation might also be present. No changes in the *ENG* sequence were detected.

Genetic analysis found a change in heterozygous condition in *ACVRL1/ALK1*, in the splicing consensus, after exon 4: c.525 + 1G > T (Figure 1), being the first time that this mutation has been described. Figure 1 shows the sequence of the mutated region in the proband (A) and the corresponding wild-type region in a healthy relative (B).

Once the mutation in the index case was known, the family decided to collect samples from all their relatives who intended to be genetically diagnosed. The samples (buccal swaps) were then sent to our lab in Madrid for diagnosis.

These samples are included in a Peruvian family pedigree showing HHT symptoms (Figure 2). Of these, a total of 24 samples were analyzed for the presence of the mutation found in the index case. Among them, 10 out of the 24 presented the mutation in a heterozygous condition.

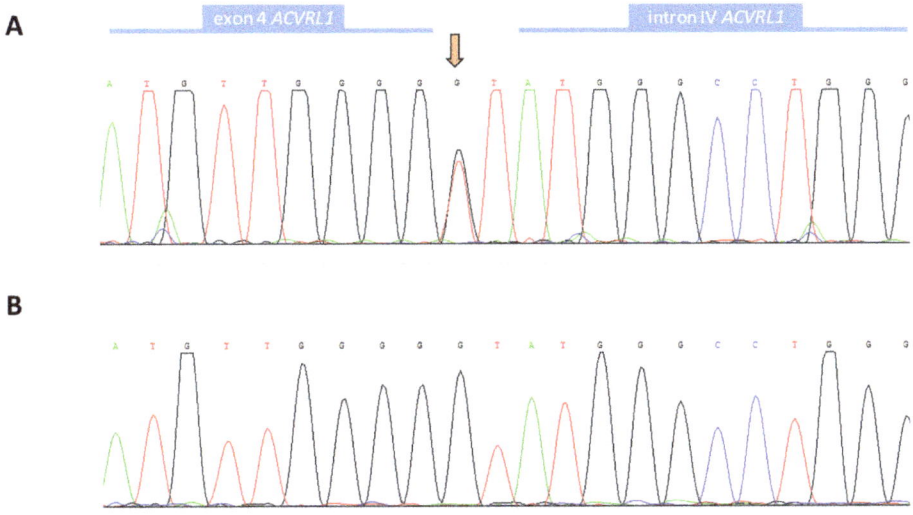

Figure 1. Normal (**B**) and mutated (**A**) exon 4-intron IV boundary sequences of the *ACVRL1/ALK1* gene. These sequences were obtained with a forward primer with the Chromas software.

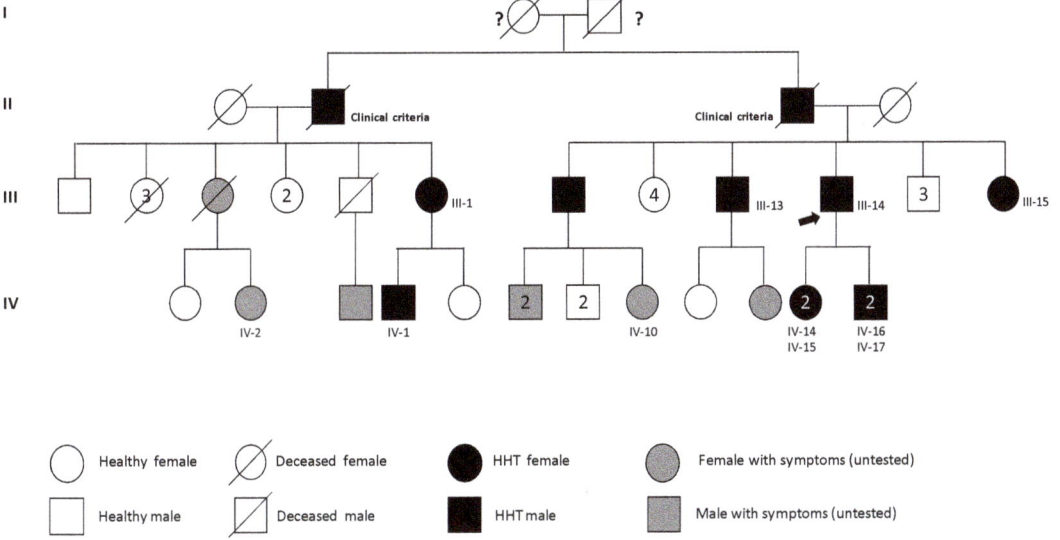

Figure 2. Pedigree of the affected family. In black, individuals with reported HHT (positive for mutation), in open, individuals with no HHT symptoms (negative for mutation) and in grey individuals with HHT clinical symptoms but untested. The black arrow indicates the proband. Numbers inside the symbols indicates the number of siblings with same phenotype. (**I–IV** indicate the family generations).

3.2. Clinical Symptoms

Table 2 shows the clinical symptoms of the positive-for-HHT family members. In general, the symptoms are as expected for HHT type 2, in which the vascular lesions are more related to the gastrointestinal tract [14], as shown by the clinical report of telangiectasias in both the stomach and colon. In two cases, liver screening was performed and revealed the presence of HAVM.

Table 2. Clinical symptoms of the family members with Curaçao criteria (* indicates index case, F: female, M: male).

Patient	Sex	Age	Epistaxis	Telangiectases	Avms	Screening	Other Diseases
III-1	F	64	yes	Face, fingers	—	none	not referred
III-13	M	69	yes	Back, face, fingers, legs, tongue,	gastric, colon	gastrointestinal endoscopy, colonoscopy	Gastric metaplasia, Anemia
III-14 *	M	65	yes	Face, fingers, Tongue	gastric, colon, liver	gastrointestinal (endoscopy, colonoscopy), brain, lung, liver,	not referred
III-15	M	64	yes	Face, fingers, gums, tongue	gastric	Gastric endoscopy	Parkinson/PVI
IV-1	M	38	yes	Not detected	none	not screened	not referred
IV-2	F	32	yes	Tongue	none	not screened	not referred
IV-10	F	49	yes	Face, fingers, lips, tongue	liver, colon	Colonoscopy, liver	not referred
IV-14	F	35	yes	Face, fingers, tongue	none	not screened	not referred
IV-15	F	28	yes	Not detected	none	not screened	not referred
IV-16	M	26	yes	Chest, face, fingers, tongue	none	not screened	not referred
IV-17	M	40	yes	Fingers	none	not screened	not referred

Screening for pulmonary and cerebral AVMs was not performed in most cases. Therefore, we cannot discard the occurrence of PAVMs or cerebral arteriovenous malformations (CAVMs) in some patients, although they would be asymptomatic. Indeed, anemia, a consequence of nosebleeds and of gastrointestinal bleeding, is a symptom present in the older patients.

3.3. RNA Expression Levels of ACVRL1 and ENG in Macrophages

Figure 3 shows the RNA expression of *ACVRL1/ALK1* in the patient compared to a healthy relative. *ENG* expression was also analyzed, since both ENG and ALK1 proteins participate in the TGFβ/BMP9 receptor complex. As described in Section 2.3, RNA expression was analyzed by quantitative PCR in attached cells (PBMCs), mainly macrophages [15,16], which express *ENG* and *ACVRL1/ALK1*. The amount of RNA was normalized to the amount of 18S RNA as a housekeeping gene.

Figure 3 shows the normalized RNA expression levels of *ENG* and *ACVRL1/ALK1* of the proband. While the expression level of *ACVRL1/ALK1* is not significantly different between the proband and healthy control, *ENG* is significantly decreased in the former. It should be stressed that the mutation occurring in *ALK1/ACVRL1* is located at the splice site and, in principle, does not affect the amount of mRNA. On the contrary, the change in *ENG* expression may be a consequence of a transcriptional regulation, in response to decreased functional levels of ALK1.

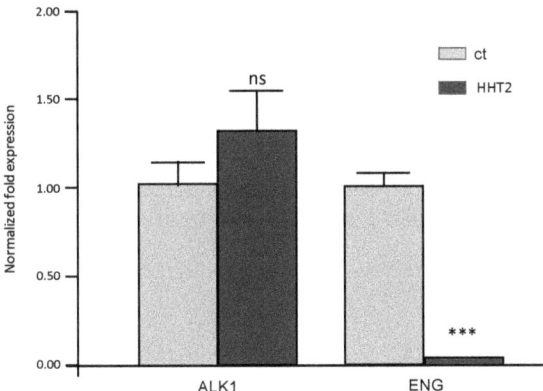

Figure 3. RT-qPCR of ALK1 in the HHT proband (HHT2) and unaffected relative (ct), showing the quantification of ALK1 RNA (ns: *non-significant*; *** $p < 0.005$).

3.4. Isolation of RNA Containing Intron IV of ACVRL1/ALK1 in the Proband

Since the mutation found in this Peruvian family affects the guanine nucleobase belonging to the splicing consensus signal placed at +1 downstream of the exon 4 of *ACVRL1/ALK1*, this change would lead to the inclusion of intron IV in part of the transcripts from the mutated allele in the proband, whereas in the wild-type allele, intron IV would not be present. The presence of the intron would lead to a premature stop codon in translation in half of the transcripts. The stop codon is predicted to be immediately after intron IV, in the first codon of exon 5. Therefore, translation would proceed 48 amino acids within intron IV after exon 4.

To demonstrate the presence of an abnormal transcript, total RNA was isolated from the proband and a healthy relative. The RNA was then retrotranscribed and used as a template for PCR amplification using as forward primer that knots within exon 4 but near the exon 4/intron IV boundary, and as reverse, a primer that knots within exon 5 near intron IV of the ACVRL1/ALK1 gene, as shown in Figure 4A. After PCR, the amplified DNA fragments were as shown in Figure 4B. The expected fragment size when intron IV is removed would be 68 bp; however, if intron IV was included (203 bp), another fragment larger than 250 bp would be detected. In Figure 4B, we can see that in lane 2 (healthy control), only a fragment of less than 100 bp is detected. However, in the case of the proband, two fragments could be detected, one of the same size as in lane 2, and one higher up, above the 250 bp size marker. These data conformed to our expectation that the larger fragment represented the RNA with the intron IV incorporated.

To demonstrate that the large fragment contained the intron IV, the DNA fragment was eluted and subjected to Sanger sequencing using the same reverse primer species used for DNA amplification. The sequencing result revealed the presence of the whole intron in this fragment, as shown in Figure 4C.

In conclusion, the evidence reported here strongly suggests that the mutation found is directly responsible for a splicing failure in around half of the transcripts, which will include intron IV of *ACVRL1/ALK1* gene and will generate a premature translation stop in ALK1 synthesis. Thus, the phenotype will be one of haploinsufficiency in those cells expressing ALK1, mainly endothelial cells.

A

```
ccacccaacctccttcggagcagccgggaacagatggccagctggccctgatcctgggccccgtgctggccttgc
tggccctggtggccctgggtgtcctgggcctgtggcatgtccgacggaggcaggagaagcagcgtggcctgcaca
gcgagctgggagagtccagtctcatcctgaaagcatctgagcagggcgacagcatgttggggtatgggcctgggg
acctgggacacagggtgtaggaggggcagataggaactgcagaatcagaggggtcacccagagattagagccggt
ggggagctgggcgagtgaggagcttgcagtgacccagcaggtcccaggtcgaggatagagaaggggctgtggct
ggttgtggcagcctctcagtggcctctccgtaccccaggacctcctggacagtgactgcaccacagggagtggc
tcagggctccccttcctggtgcagaggacagtggcacggcaggttgccttggtggagtgtgtgg
```

Fwd ex4 5'-3' gcatgtccgacggaggca
Rev ex5 5'-3' ccacacactccaccaaggc

B

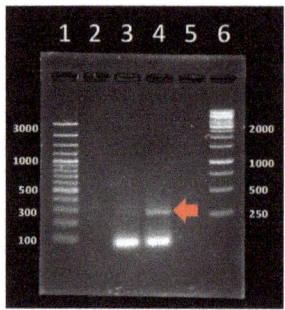

C

```
agcgagctgggagagtccagtctcatcctgaaagcatctgagcaggg
cgacagcatgttggggtatgggcctggggacctgggacacagggtgt
aggaggggcagataggaactgcagaatcagaggggtcacccagagat
tagagccggtggggagctgggcgagtgaggagcttgcagtgacccag
caggtcccaggtcgaggatagagaaggggctgtggctggttgtggc
agcctctcagtggcctctccgtaccccaggacctcctggacagtga
ctgcacc
```

Figure 4. (**A**) DNA sequence of the terminal part of exon 4, intron IV and the beginning of exon 5 of the ACVRL1/ALK1 gene. Sequence of the forward and reverse primers used for PCR amplification show the alignment region within this DNA sequence. (**B**) PCR of the cDNA from HHT and unaffected relative showing, in the case of HHT, the presence of an abnormal band > 250 bp corresponding to the species containing intron IV of ALK1 (highlighted by a red arrow). (**C**) Sequence of exon 4 border and intron IV of ALK1 obtained from the >250 bp band shown in B. Marker sizes are shown.

4. Discussion

This work presents a new mutation in *ACVRL1/ALK1* as a cause of HHT2, in a large family from Peru, although not all of them have been genetically analyzed. A previous paper [17] described the presence of a novel mutation found in exon 4 of the *ENG* gene c.408delA, at amino acid residue 136, found in four affected members of a family from Peru. However, after this report, and to the best of our knowledge, this manuscript reports the results of the largest cohort of HHT ever published in Peru.

The work is also remarkable, as an example of international, cross-border cooperation, so necessary in rare diseases, where it is difficult to find specialized centers and research on them, especially in areas with fewer resources, as would be the case for HHT and Peru. Taking into account the difficulties in the diagnoses of rare diseases, we turn to clinicians and researchers in developed countries to collaborate and help in the diagnoses, follow-up, and treatments of patients with rare diseases in developing countries. The procedure described here is fast, easy, and feasible.

The cooperation began with the visit to Spain of the index case, diagnosed at the National Institute of Neoplasic diseases in Lima, Peru, as a patient with HHT, following Curaçao criteria. Clinical care included treatment with an ENT specialist in HHT and a clinician of reference in the treatment of epistaxis in HHT, by applying the sclerotherapy technique [13]. Clinical care was also completed with a visit to internal medicine for the detection of possible AVMs in internal organs.

At the same time, genetic diagnosis of the patient was carried out, starting with amplification and Sanger sequencing of the exons and intron–exon boundaries of the *ACVRL1/ALK1* gene, due to the patient's clinical data. The absence of PAVMs and the presence of nasal, gastric bleeding and HAVMs suggested a higher possibility for having an *ACVRL1/ALK1* mutation. Indeed, a mutation not previously described in the literature was found in c.525 + 1G > T, at the consensus splice site after exon 4. The variant could be classified "a priori" as pathogenic, following the American College of Medical Genetics and Genomics (ACMG) guidelines [18]. In fact, the familial concordance study establishes a strong basis, as individuals III-13, III-14 (proband), and III-15 all had the mutation and met the clinical diagnostic criteria. Moreover, two additional pathogenic variants are known in the same locus (c.525 + 1G > C; c.5252 + 1G > A).

Subsequently, once the bioethics and biosafety measures had been approved, a total of 24 family members residing in Peru underwent genetic analysis. The samples were taken with buccal swaps, which were sent to Spain. Thus, 9 of the 25 relatives were genetically diagnosed as heterozygous carriers of the mutation. The clinical phenotypes were analyzed, within the limitations found due to the dispersion of the affected members in different parts of Peru, and not in the hospital in Lima, where the index case was diagnosed. The clinical symptomatology found makes it desirable that family members with genetic diagnosis of HHT can be followed up by the physician of the National Institute of Neoplasic diseases in Lima, and that a reference unit of HHT for Peru could be created at this hospital.

On the other hand, on the more molecular side, the presence in heterozygosis of this c.525 + 1G > T variant suggested that there would not be correct splicing between exons 4 and 5 of *ACVRL1/ALK1*. A deficiency in the *ACVRL1/ALK1* messenger would not be expected, since in principle, transcription would proceed, although subsequent splicing would be aberrant. Figure 3 shows that there were no significant differences between ALK1 transcript levels in the proband compared to a normal relative. It is also remarkable to see how the amount of *ENG* transcript is downregulated in the proband vs. control. This deficit can be explained because there is a coordinated transcriptional regulation between *ENG* and *ACVRL1/ALK1* described by our group [11,19,20]. Since both ENG and ALK1 proteins are present in the TGF-β/BMP9 signaling complex, when there is a deficit in the ALK1 protein, a negative feedback occurs in ENG transcription, so that at the protein level, the signaling complex is balanced [11,20], thus, adapting to the ALK1 deficit scenario. Different authors in Europe and the United States have made contributions of genotype–phenotype correlations [21–23].

As demonstrated in Figure 4, aberrant splicing leads to the inclusion of intron IV in half of the transcripts—those originating from the transcript of the mutated allele. From total RNA isolation, an anomalous RNA species is detected only in the proband. Sequencing of this species confirmed the presence of exons 4 and 5, along with the presence of the intron between them. This aberrant splice variant would result in a premature termination codon, which would not result in a functional protein.

The limitation of this study is the lack of enough biological material, either endothelial cells [19] or macrophages, to perform protein studies to see the amount and type of ALK1 species in both the mutated case and in the healthy family member. In addition, with a primary endothelial cell culture, the amount of surface protein could be analyzed by flow cytometry in comparison with a healthy control. Finally, various experiments, including TGF-β/BMP9 pathway-dependent signaling and functional experiments mentioned above, could be performed.

5. Conclusions

- A new mutation in the *ACVRL1/ALK1* gene (HHT2), involving the consensus splice junction immediately after exon 4, c.525 + 1G > T, was found in a member of a large Peruvian family with a history of HHT-compatible symptoms.
- Among 25 members of this family, 10 of them showed the presence of the mutation in a heterozygous condition, while 15 showed the wild-type alleles. The pres-

- ence of this mutation was correlated with the clinical symptoms of HHT following Curaçao criteria.
- It has been demonstrated that the mutation leads to an abnormal splicing of *ACVRL1/ALK1* intron IV, since an RNA species containing exon4-intron IV-exon 5 was isolated, in addition to normal splicing in around half of the transcripts in an affected member.
- We strongly recommend the screening and follow up of the affected members according to the clinical guidelines of HHT.
- This manuscript may contribute to the awareness of HHT in Peru and to the creation of a reference center together with the patient association, for this rare disease in Peru.

Author Contributions: Conceptualization, S.E.D., V.A., A.M.C. and L.M.B.; methodology, M.P., L.R.-P., S.V. and J.P.P.; software, V.A. and M.P.; validation, S.E.D., V.A. and L.M.B.; formal analysis, V.A., S.E.D., M.P. and L.M.B.; investigation, S.V., J.P.P., S.E.D., L.R.-P., V.A. and M.P.; resources, S.V., J.P.P. and S.E.D.; writing—original draft preparation, V.A., M.P. and L.M.B.; writing—review and editing, V.A., M.P., J.C.-V., A.M.C. and L.M.B.; funding acquisition, L.M.B. All authors have read and agreed to the published version of the manuscript.

Funding: This research was funded by MINECO (Ministry of Economy of Spain), grant number SAF2017-83351R, and by MICINN (Ministry of Science and Innovation of Spain), grant number PID2020-115371RB-I00. LR-P was the recipient of a contract from an internal project of CSIC (PIE201820E073).

Institutional Review Board Statement: The study was conducted in accordance with the Declaration of Helsinki and approved by the Institutional Review Board (Human Ethics Committee) of CSIC (National Research Council of Spain) for studies involving humans (protocol code 075 at 2017).

Informed Consent Statement: Written informed consent was obtained from the patient(s) to publish this paper.

Data Availability Statement: Data supporting the reported results can be found in our laboratory records. DNA and RNA are part of the collection associated with the research of the group.

Acknowledgments: We acknowledge the support given by Sol Marcos (MD) reference ENT for HHT disease at HUFA. We also are indebted to all the patients from Peru who contributed their samples to the genetic analysis and, with their informed consent, to the diagnosis and publication of data.

Conflicts of Interest: The authors declare no conflict of interest.

References

1. Shovlin, C.L. Hereditary haemorrhagic telangiectasia: Pathophysiology, diagnosis and treatment. *Blood Rev.* **2010**, *24*, 203–219. [CrossRef] [PubMed]
2. Faughnan, M.E.; Palda, V.A.; Garcia-Tsao, G.; Geisthoff, U.W.; McDonald, J.; Proctor, D.D.; Spears, J.; Brown, D.H.; Buscarini, E.; Chesnutt, M.S.; et al. International guidelines for the diagnosis and management of hereditary haemorrhagic telangiectasia. *J. Med. Genet.* **2011**, *48*, 73–87. [CrossRef] [PubMed]
3. McDonald, J.; Bayrak-Toydemir, P.; Pyeritz, R.E. Hereditary hemorrhagic telangiectasia: An overview of diagnosis, management, and pathogenesis. *Genet. Med.* **2011**, *13*, 607–616. [CrossRef]
4. McDonald, J.; Wooderchak-Donahue, W.; VanSant Webb, C.; Whitehead, K.; Stevenson, D.A.; Bayrak-Toydemir, P. Hereditary hemorrhagic telangiectasia: Genetics and molecular diagnostics in a new era. *Front. Genet.* **2015**, *6*, 1. [CrossRef] [PubMed]
5. Faughnan, M.E.; Mager, J.J.; Hetts, S.W.; Palda, V.A.; Lang-Robertson, K.; Buscarini, E.; Deslandres, E.; Kasthuri, R.S.; Lausman, A.; Poetker, D.; et al. Second international guidelines for the diagnosis and management of hereditary hemorrhagic telangiectasia. *Ann. Intern. Med.* **2021**, *174*, 1035–1036. [CrossRef] [PubMed]
6. Richards-Yutz, J.; Grant, K.; Chao, E.C.; Walther, S.E.; Ganguly, A. Update on molecular diagnosis of hereditary hemorrhagic telangiectasia. *Hum. Genet.* **2010**, *128*, 61–77. [CrossRef] [PubMed]
7. Cole, S.G.; Begbie, M.E.; Wallace, G.M.F.; Shovlin, C.L.L. A new locus for hereditary haemorrhagic telangiectasia (HHT3) maps to chromosome 5. *J. Med. Genet.* **2005**, *42*, 577–582. [CrossRef]
8. Bayrak-Toydemir, P.; McDonald, J.; Akarsu, N.; Toydemir, R.M.; Calderon, F.; Tuncali, T.; Tang, W.; Miller, F.; Mao, R. A fourth locus for hereditary hemorrhagic telangiectasia maps to chromosome 7. *Am. J. Med. Genet. A* **2006**, *140*, 2155–2162. [CrossRef]
9. Wooderchak-Donahue, W.L.; McDonald, J.; O'Fallon, B.; Upton, P.D.; Li, W.; Roman, B.L.; Young, S.; Plant, P.; Fülöp, G.T.; Langa, C.; et al. BMP9 mutations cause a vascular-anomaly syndrome with phenotypic overlap with hereditary hemorrhagic telangiectasia. *Am. J. Hum. Genet.* **2013**, *93*, 530–537. [CrossRef]

10. Gallione, C.; Aylsworth, A.S.; Beis, J.; Berk, T.; Bernhardt, B.; Clark, R.D.; Clericuzio, C.; Danesino, C.; Drautz, J.; Fahl, J.; et al. Overlapping spectra of SMAD4 mutations in juvenile polyposis (JP) and JP-HHT syndrome. *Am. J. Med. Genet. A* **2010**, *152A*, 333–339. [CrossRef]
11. Fernandez-L, A.; Sanz-Rodriguez, F.; Zarrabeitia, R.; Perez-Molino, A.; Morales, C.; Restrepo, C.M.; Ramirez, J.R.; Coto, E.; Lenato, G.M.; Bernabeu, C.; et al. Mutation study of spanish patients with hereditary hemorrhagic telangiectasia and expression analysis of endoglin and ALK1. *Hum. Mutat.* **2006**, *27*, 295. [CrossRef] [PubMed]
12. Sanger, F.; Air, G.M.; Barrell, B.G.; Brown, N.L.; Coulson, A.R.; Fiddes, J.C.; Hutchison, C.A.; Slocombe, P.M.; Smith, M. Nucleotide sequence of bacteriophage φx174 DNA. *Nature* **1977**, *265*, 687–695. [CrossRef] [PubMed]
13. Marcos, S.; Botella, L.M.; Albiñana, V.; Arbia, A.; de Rosales, A.M. Sclerotherapy on demand with polidocanol to treat hht nosebleeds. *J. Clin. Med.* **2021**, *10*, 3845. [CrossRef] [PubMed]
14. Ruiz-Llorente, L.; Gallardo-Vara, E.; Rossi, E.; Smadja, D.M.; Botella, L.M.; Bernabeu, C. Endoglin and alk1 as therapeutic targets for hereditary hemorrhagic telangiectasia. *Expert Opin. Ther. Targets* **2017**, *21*, 933–947. [CrossRef]
15. Lastres, P.; Bellon, T.; Cabañas, C.; Sanchez-Madrid, F.; Acevedo, A.; Gougos, A.; Letarte, M.; Bernabeu, C. Regulated expression on human macrophages of endoglin, an Arg-Gly-Asp-containing surface antigen. *Eur. J. Immunol.* **1992**, *22*, 393–397. [CrossRef]
16. Sanz-Rodriguez, F.; Fernandez-L, A.; Zarrabeitia, R.; Perez-Molino, A.; Ramírez, J.R.; Coto, E.; Bernabeu, C.; Botella, L.M. Mutation analysis in Spanish patients with hereditary hemorrhagic telangiectasia: Deficient endoglin up-regulation in activated monocytes. *Clin. Chem.* **2004**, *50*, 2003–2011. [CrossRef]
17. Zevallos-Morales, A.; Murillo, A.; Dueñas-Roque, M.M.; Prötzel, A.; Venegas-Tresierra, L.; Ángeles-Villalba, V.; Guevara-Cruz, M.; Chávez-Gil, A.; Fujita, R.; Guevara-Fujita, M.L. Novel mutation in ENG gene causing hereditary hemorrhagic telangiectasia in a peruvian family. *Genet. Mol. Biol.* **2020**, *43*, e20190126. [CrossRef]
18. Richards, S.; Aziz, N.; Bale, S.; Bick, D.; Das, S.; Gastier-Foster, J.; Grody, W.W.; Hegde, M.; Lyon, E.; Spector, E.; et al. Standards and guidelines for the interpretation of sequence variants: A joint consensus recommendation of the American College of Medical Genetics and Genomics and the Association for Molecular Pathology. *Genet. Med.* **2015**, *17*, 405–424. [CrossRef]
19. Fernandez-L, A.; Sanz-Rodriguez, F.; Zarrabeitia, R.; Pérez-Molino, A.; Hebbel, R.P.; Nguyen, J.; Bernabéu, C.; Botella, L.M. Blood outgrowth endothelial cells from Hereditary Haemorrhagic Telangiectasia patients reveal abnormalities compatible with vascular lesions. *Cardiovasc. Res.* **2005**, *68*, 235–248. [CrossRef]
20. Fernández-L, A.; Sanz-Rodriguez, F.; Blanco, F.J.; Bernabéu, C.; Botella, L.M. Hereditary hemorrhagic telangiectasia, a vascular dysplasia affecting the TGF-β signaling pathway. *Clin. Med. Res.* **2006**, *4*, 66–78. [CrossRef]
21. Letteboer, T.G.; Mager, J.J.; Snijder, R.J.; Koeleman, B.P.; Lindhout, D.; Ploos van Amstel, J.K.; Westermann, C.J. Genotype-phenotype relationship in hereditary haemorrhagic telangiectasia. *J. Med. Genet.* **2006**, *43*, 371–377.
22. Bayrak-Toydemir, P.; McDonald, J.; Markewitz, B.; Lewin, S.; Miller, F.; Chou, L.S.; Gedge, F.; Tang, W.; Coon, H.; Mao, R. Genotype-phenotype correlation in hereditary hemorrhagic telangiectasia: Mutations and manifestations. *Am. J. Med. Genet. A* **2006**, *140*, 463–470. [CrossRef] [PubMed]
23. Lesca, G.; Olivieri, C.; Burnichon, N.; Pagella, F.; Carette, M.F.; Gilbert-Dussardier, B.; Goizet, C.; Roume, J.; Rabilloud, M.; Saurin, J.C.; et al. Genotype-phenotype correlations in hereditary hemorrhagic telangiectasia: Data from the French-Italian HHT network. *Genet. Med.* **2007**, *9*, 14–22. [CrossRef] [PubMed]

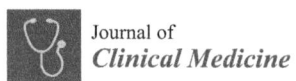

Article

Distribution of Cerebrovascular Phenotypes According to Variants of the *ENG* and *ACVRL1* Genes in Subjects with Hereditary Hemorrhagic Telangiectasia

Eleonora Gaetani [1,2,*], Elisabetta Peppucci [1,3], Fabiana Agostini [1,2], Luigi Di Martino [1,2], Emanuela Lucci Cordisco [1,4], Carmelo L. Sturiale [1,3], Alfredo Puca [1,3], Angelo Porfidia [1,2], Andrea Alexandre [1,5], Alessandro Pedicelli [1,5] and Roberto Pola [1,2]

- [1] HHT Center, Fondazione Policlinico Universitario A. Gemelli IRCCS, Università Cattolica del Sacro Cuore, 00168 Rome, Italy; elisabetta.peppucci@gmail.com (E.P.); fabiana.agostini@libero.it (F.A.); luigidimartino7@gmail.com (L.D.M.); emanuela.luccicordisco@policlinicogemelli.it (E.L.C.); carmelo.sturiale@policlinicogemelli.it (C.L.S.); alfredo.puca@policlinicogemelli.it (A.P.); angelo.porfidia@policlinicogemelli.it (A.P.); andrea.alexandre@policlinicogemelli.it (A.A.); alessandro.pedicelli@policlinicogemelli.it (A.P.); roberto.pola@unicatt.it (R.P.)
- [2] Department of Medicine, Fondazione Policlinico Universitario A. Gemelli IRCCS, Università Cattolica del Sacro Cuore, 00168 Rome, Italy
- [3] Department of Neurosurgery, Fondazione Policlinico Universitario A. Gemelli IRCCS, Università Cattolica del Sacro Cuore, 00168 Rome, Italy
- [4] Department of Genetics, Fondazione Policlinico Universitario A. Gemelli IRCCS, Università Cattolica del Sacro Cuore, 00168 Rome, Italy
- [5] Department of Radiology, Fondazione Policlinico Universitario A. Gemelli IRCCS, Università Cattolica del Sacro Cuore, 00168 Rome, Italy
- * Correspondence: eleonora.gaetani@unicatt.it

Abstract: Hereditary Hemorrhagic Telangiectasia (HHT) is an autosomal dominant disorder caused, in more than 80% of cases, by mutations of either the endoglin (*ENG*) or the activin A receptor-like type 1 (*ACVRL1*) gene. Several hundred variants have been identified in these HHT-causing genes, including deletions, missense and nonsense mutations, splice defects, duplications, and insertions. In this study, we have analyzed retrospectively collected images of magnetic resonance angiographies (MRA) of the brain of HHT patients, followed at the HHT Center of our University Hospital, and looked for the distribution of cerebrovascular phenotypes according to specific gene variants. We found that cerebrovascular malformations were heterogeneous among HHT patients, with phenotypes that ranged from classical arteriovenous malformations (AVM) to intracranial aneurysms (IA), developmental venous anomalies (DVA), and cavernous angiomas (CA). There was also wide heterogeneity among the variants of the *ENG* and *ACVRL1* genes, which included known pathogenic variants, variants of unknown significance, variants pending classification, and variants which had not been previously reported. The percentage of patients with cerebrovascular malformations was significantly higher among subjects with *ENG* variants than *ACVRL1* variants (25.0% vs. 13.1%, $p < 0.05$). The prevalence of neurovascular anomalies was different among subjects with different gene variants, with an incidence that ranged from 3.3% among subjects with the c.1231C > T, c.200G > A, or c.1120C > T missense mutations of the *ACVRL1* gene, to 75.0% among subjects with the c.1435C > T missense mutation of the *ACVRL1* gene. Further studies and larger sample sizes are required to confirm these findings.

Keywords: hereditary hemorrhagic telangiectasia; cerebrovascular malformations; arteriovenous malformations; genetics; gene variants; *ENG*; *ACVRL1*

Citation: Gaetani, E.; Peppucci, E.; Agostini, F.; Di Martino, L.; Lucci Cordisco, E.; Sturiale, C.L.; Puca, A.; Porfidia, A.; Alexandre, A.; Pedicelli, A.; et al. Distribution of Cerebrovascular Phenotypes According to Variants of the *ENG* and *ACVRL1* Genes in Subjects with Hereditary Hemorrhagic Telangiectasia. *J. Clin. Med.* 2022, 11, 2685. https://doi.org/10.3390/jcm11102685

Academic Editor: Angel M. Cuesta

Received: 7 April 2022
Accepted: 5 May 2022
Published: 10 May 2022

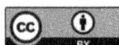

Copyright: © 2022 by the authors. Licensee MDPI, Basel, Switzerland. This article is an open access article distributed under the terms and conditions of the Creative Commons Attribution (CC BY) license (https://creativecommons.org/licenses/by/4.0/).

1. Introduction

Hereditary hemorrhagic telangiectasia (HHT) is a rare autosomal dominant genetic disorder with an estimated prevalence of 1–5 cases/10,000 individuals [1]. The clinical hallmarks of the disease are multiple arteriovenous shunts, or arteriovenous malformations (AVMs), affecting several organs, including the skin, nasal and oral mucosa, lungs, liver, brain, and gastrointestinal tract [2,3].

Most HHT-causing variants are detected in endoglin (*ENG*) and activin A receptor type II-like kinase 1 (*ALK1/ACVRL1*) genes [4–6]. Less than 2% of cases are instead due to variants of the Family Member 4 (*SMAD4*) gene [7]. Pathogenic variants in the *ENG* and *ACVRL1* genes result in different HHT types, commonly referred to as HHT1 and HHT2, respectively [4,5] Pathogenic variants in the *SMAD4* gene give rise to a combined syndrome of HHT and juvenile polyposis (JP): the JP-HHT syndrome [7]. Several hundred variants of the *ENG* and *ACVRL1* genes, including deletions, duplications, missense and nonsense mutations, splice defects, and silent variants, have been identified in patients with HHT [8,9] and are present in HHT mutation databases (http://arup.utah.edu/database/ENG/ENG_welcome.php, accessed on 7 March 2022) [10]. Whether single gene variants are associated with specific HHT phenotypes is under investigation and remains to be determined, since HHT is a rare disease and many of the above-mentioned gene variants have been reported in the literature only once.

At the level of the central nervous system (CNS), there is a wide spectrum of possible cerebrovascular malformations in HHT. These include AVMs, but also cavernous malformations (CAs), capillary telangiectasias (CTs), developmental venous anomalies (DVAs), arteriovenous fistulas (AVFs), and intracranial aneurysms (IAs) [11,12].

The aim of this study was to assess the distribution of different types of cerebrovascular malformations according to specific variants of the *ENG* and *ACVRL1* genes in subjects with HHT.

2. Materials and Methods

Ethics. This study was approved by the Ethics Committee of the Fondazione Policlinico Universitario A. Gemelli IRCCS (protocol number 6241/20, ID 2999, date of approval 20 February 2020). Due to the retrospective nature of the study, and the fact that the study only consisted of analysis of data available in the electronic database of our hospital, additional informed consent was not required.

Patients. We collected data of patients followed at the HHT Center of the Fondazione Policlinico Universitario A. Gemelli IRCCS of Rome, Italy. Only data of patients who had a genetically established diagnosis of HHT and had undergone Magnetic Resonance Imaging of the brain with angiographic study (MRA) were collected.

Review of MRA. MRA images were reviewed by four independent investigators of our HHT Center (two neuroradiologists and two neurosurgeons), blinded to the genotypes of patients. The results of the review were tabulated as follows: negative exam (no evidence of cerebrovascular malformations); positive exams (evidence of at least one of the following cerebrovascular malformations: AVM, CA, CT, DVA, AVF, IA).

Statistical analysis. Results are presented as mean ± SD or number and percentage. Comparisons between groups were made by using Student's t test. Differences were considered statistically significant for $p < 0.05$.

3. Results

We identified 77 patients with genetically verified HHT with fully accessible MRA images of the brain, which is part of the screening routinely performed on HHT patients at our center. The demographic, clinical, genetic, and neuroradiological characteristics of these patients are reported in Table 1. Briefly, all patients were Italians of Caucasian ancestry. Mean age was 53.6 ± 16.7 years. Male/female ratio was 33/44. Most patients (98.7%) belonged to a definite HHT family, while only one patient (1.3%) had negative family history. Regarding HHT clinical hallmarks, recurrent epistaxis and cutaneous telangiectasias were present in 94.8% and 90.9% of patients, respectively. Lung and liver involvement was found in 32.5% and 44.1% of patients, respectively. GI bleeding was reported in 24.7% of cases. *ENG* and *ACVRL1* variants were found in 16 (20.8%) and

61 (79.2%) patients, respectively. MRAs were negative for any type of cerebrovascular malformations in 65 patients (84.4%), while they were positive in 12 patients (15.6%), with a male/female ratio of 5/7. There were four patients (three males and one female) with an AVM, three patients (one male and two females) with an IA, one patient (male) with the concomitant presence of an AVM and an IA, two patients (2 females) with a CA, and two patients (two females) with a DVA, for a total of 13 vascular malformations.

Table 1. Characteristics of the study population.

Mean age (years±SD)	53.6 ± 16.7
Gender (male/female ratio)	33/44
Epistaxis (n/total)	73/77
Mucocutaneous telangiectases (n/total)	70/77
Family history of HHT (n/total)	76/77
Pulmonary AVMs (n/total)	25/77
Hepatic AVMs (n/total)	34/77
Gastrointestinal AVMs (n/total)	19/77
Cerebrovascular malformations (n/total) - Arteriovenous malformation (AVM) - Intracranial aneurysm (IA) - Developmental venous anomaly (DVA) - Cavernous angioma (CA) - AVM + IA	12/77 4/12 3/12 2/12 2/12 1/12
ENG mutations *ACVRL1* mutations	16/77 61/77

A schematic representation of the diverse types of cerebrovascular malformations found in our cohort is shown in Figure 1.

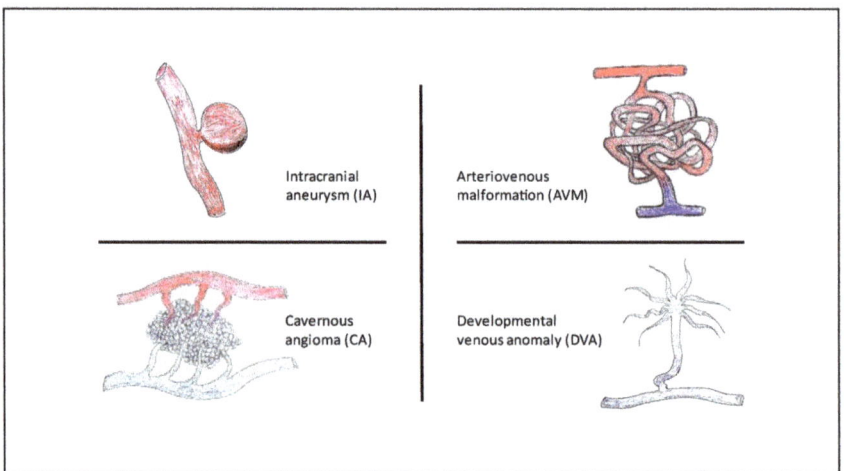

Figure 1. Types of cerebrovascular malformations found in our cohort of HHT patients.

Figure 2 presents instead representative MR images of the diverse types of cerebrovascular malformations found in our HHT cohort.

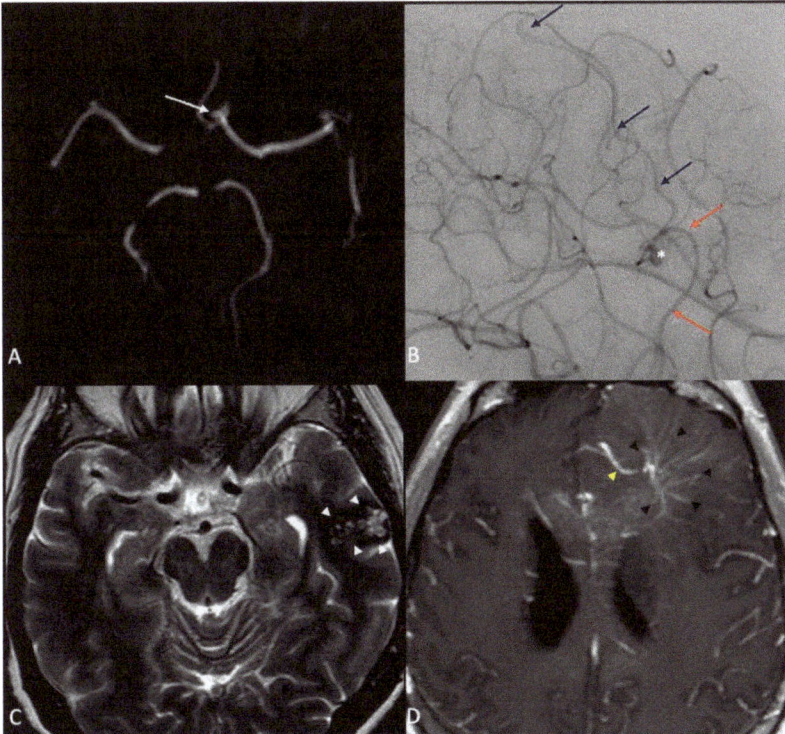

Figure 2. Representative MR images of the cerebrovascular malformations found in our cohort. (**A**) 3D-time of flight MR demonstrating a small anterior communicating artery aneurysm. (**B**) Lateral projection in a Digital Subtraction Angiography during internal carotid artery injection: a small nidus of an arteriovenous malformation (AVM) is evident (white asterisk), as well as an arterial feeder coming from the middle cerebral artery (red arrows) and the draining vein going to the superior sagittal sinus (blue arrows). (**C**) MR T2-weighted axial image shows a large, cavernous angioma (CA) in the cortical region of the left temporal lobe (white arrow heads), with a characteristic "popcorn" appearance and a rim of signal loss due to hemosiderin. (**D**) MR T1-weghted post-contrast axial image showing a vascular malformation characterized by a "caput medusae" (black arrowheads), which is a collection of dilated medullary veins, which converges in an enlarged transcortical or collector vein (yellow arrowhead), which is pathognomonic of developmental venous anomaly (DVA).

Table 2 reports the different gene variants that we found in our cohort. In total, there were 10 *ENG* variants and 24 *ACVRL1* variants. Among the *ENG* variants, seven were known pathogenic variants (which were found in a total of 13 patients), one was a variant pending classification, and two were variants not previously reported in the HHT mutation database. Among the *ACVRL1* variants, 11 were known pathogenic variants (distributed in a total of 45 patients), three were variants pending classification (distributed in a total of three patients), one was a variant of unknown significance (VUS), and eight were variants not previously reported in the HHT mutation database (distributed in a total of 11 patients). The most represented gene variants in our population were the c.1231C > T (14 patients from five unrelated families), the c.200G > A (eight patients from three unrelated families), and the c.1120C > T (eight patients from three unrelated families) missense mutations of the *ACVRL1* gene.

Table 3 reports the distribution of cerebrovascular malformations according to *ENG* and *ACVRL1* variants. The percentage of patients with cerebrovascular malformations was significantly higher among subjects with ENG variants (four out of 16 patients) than among subjects with ACVRL1 variants (eight out of 61 patients) (25.0% vs. 13.1%, respectively, $p < 0.05$). Among the four patients with ENG variants who had cerebrovascular malformations, three were females and one was a male. Among the eight patients with ACVRL1 variants who had cerebrovascular malformations, four were females and four were males. When the correlation analysis was limited to known pathogenic variants, the percentage of patients with cerebrovascular malformations was 23.1% in the ENG group and 11.1% in the ACVRL1 group. As mentioned above, the c.1231C > T, the c.200G > A, and the c.1120C > T missense mutations of the ACVRL1 gene were the most represented variants in our population. Taken together, they were present in 30 patients, i.e., 38.9% of the study population. However, in these 30 patients we found only one cerebrovascular anomaly, with an incidence of 3.3%. On the opposite side, there was the c.1435C > T missense mutation of the ACVRL1 gene that, although present only in four patients, was associated with three cases of cerebrovascular malformations, with an incidence of 75.0%. There was also the c.771dup variant of the ENG gene that, although found only in three patients, was associated with one case of cerebrovascular malformations (incidence 33.3%).

Table 2. Distribution of gene variants.

Nucleotide Change	Type of Variant	Classification	Patients (n)
	ENG		
c.771dup	Duplication	pathogenic	4
c.309_311del	Deletion	pathogenic	3
c.1678C > T	Nonsense	pathogenic	2
c.1199delG	Deletion	pathogenic	1
c.1 A > G	Missense	pathogenic	1
c.511C > T	Nonsense	pathogenic	1
c.967_968del	Deletion	pathogenic	1
c.1088G > A	Missense	pending classification	1
c.582_600del	deletion	not previously reported	1
c.1115T > C	Missense	not previously reported	1
	ACVRL1		
c.1231C > T	Missense	pathogenic	14
c.1120C > T	Missense	pathogenic	8
c.200G > A	Missense	pathogenic	8
c.1435C > T	Missense	pathogenic	4
c.430C > T	Missense	pathogenic	4
c.1121G > A	Missense	pathogenic	1
c.1135G > A	Missense	pathogenic	2
c.1232G > A	Missense	pathogenic	1
c.218_219insAA	Insertion	pathogenic	1
c.435del	Deletion	pathogenic	1
c.1435C > T	Missense	pathogenic	1
c.230G > A	Missense	pending classification	1
c.526G > T	Missense	pending classification	1
c.988G > T	Missense	pending classification	1
c.1445C > A	Missense	VUS	2
c.264C > G	Missense	not previously reported	2
c.847_853delinsTT	deletion-insertion	not previously reported	2
c.144_145insG	Insertion	not previously reported	1
c.771_772dup	Duplication	not previously reported	1
c.837C > G	Missense	not previously reported	1
c.1028A > C	Missense	not previously reported	1
c.398C > G	Missense	not previously reported	1
c.915_916dup	Duplication	not previously reported	1
c.738_739dup	Duplication	not previously reported	1

Table 3. Distribution of cerebrovascular malformations according to *ENG* and *ACVRL1* variants.

Nucleotide Change	Positive/Total MRA	Type of Malformation
All ENG variants	4/16 (25.0%)	
Pathogenic variants	3/13 (23.1%)	
c.1199delG	0/1 (0.0%)	–
c.1678C > T	1/2 (50.0%)	AVM
c.1A > G	1/1 (100.0%)	IA
c.309_311del	0/3 (0.0%)	–
c.511C > T	0/1 (0.0%)	–
c.771dup	1/4 (25.0%)	AVM
c.967_968del	0/1 (0.0%)	–
Other variants	1/3 (33.3%)	
c.1115T > C	1/1 (100.0%)	DVA
c.1088G > A	0/1 (0.0%)	–
c.582_600 del	0/1 (0.0%)	–
All ACVRL1 variants	8/61 (13.1%)	
Pathogenic variants	5/45 (11.1%)	
c.1120C > T	0/8 (0.0%)	–
c.1121G > A	0/1 (0.0%)	–
c.1135G > A	0/2 (0.0%)	–
c.1231C > T	1/14 (7.1%)	CA
c.1232G > A	1/1 (100.0%)	AVM + IA
c.1435C > T	3/4 (75.0%)	2 IA (M, F), 1 DVA
c.200G > A	0/8 (0.0%)	–
c.218_219insAA	0/1 (0.0%)	–
c.430C > T	0/4 (0.0%)	–
c.435del	0/1 (0.0%)	–
Other variants	3/16 (18.7%)	
c.230G > A	0/1 (0.0%)	–
c.526G > T	1/1 (100.0%)	AVM
c.988G > T	0/1 (0.0%)	–
c.1445C > A	0/2 (0.0%)	–
c.144_145insG	0/1 (0.0%)	–
c.771_772dup	1/1 (100.0%)	CA
c.837C > G	0/1 (0.0%)	–
c.1028A > C	0/1 (0.0%)	–
c.264C > G	0/2 (0.0%)	–
c.398C > G	0/1 (0.0%)	–
c.915_916dup	1/1 (100.0%)	AVM
c.847_853delinsTT	0/2 (0.0%)	–
c.738_739dup	0/1 (0.0%)	–

4. Discussion

In this study, we evaluated the distribution of cerebrovascular phenotypes according to specific *ENG* and *ACVRL1* gene variants in subjects with HHT. It is interesting to note that, in our population, neurovascular anomalies were significantly more frequent among *ENG* than *ACVRL1* patients. This is consistent with the results of a recent meta-analysis [13], showing that patients with HHT1 have a significantly higher brain AVM prevalence compared with those with HHT2 and confirms that different genetic backgrounds may have an impact on the cerebrovascular phenotypes of HHT patients.

On the other hand, it is also notable that some gene variants, although numerically well represented in our population, were never–or very rarely–associated with the presence of a cerebrovascular malformation. In particular, this was the case of the c.1231C > T, c.200G > A, and c.1120C > T missense mutations of the *ACVRL1* gene, which cumulatively were present in 24 patients (35.3% of our population) but were associated with a cerebrovascular malformation only in one case. It is also interesting that, among HHT2 patients, a consistent proportion of cerebrovascular malformations (37.5%) was found in patients carrying gene variants for which an established pathogenic role does not exist yet, according to the HHT

Mutation Database [10]. Indeed, in this study, we found nine novel variants which had never been reported previously. One of these was a deletion (c.582_600del) detected in the *ENG* gene in one patient who did not have any cerebrovascular malformation at MRA of the brain. The other eight variants which had never been reported before were in the *ACVRL1* gene and were found in a total of 10 patients. Additional studies will be important for establishing whether the relationship between these variants and cerebrovascular malformations are common or coincidental occurrences.

This study also constitutes a useful report on the incidence of cerebrovascular malformations in HHT, which was 15.6% in our population. This incidence is similar to that reported by Woodall and coll. in 2014 (18.6%) and Brinjikji and coll. in 2016 [11,14]. It is instead higher than that reported by Maher and coll. in 2001 (3.7%) [15], but it should be noted that this study took into account patients who were not screened for the presence of a cerebral vascular malformation, while our study only included subjects for whom neurovascular imaging was available. Regarding the type of malformation, our study confirms that vascular brain lesions are heterogeneous among HHT patients. AVMs were the most common in our population, with an incidence of 6.5%. IAs were also common, with an incidence of 5.2%. The notion that HHT patients often have aneurysmatic diseases has been recently confirmed by a retrospective analysis of Ring and coll., who found 43 patients with at least one aneurysm on 418 HHT subjects, with a prevalence of 10.3% [16]. Taken together, IAs and AVMs accounted for 75.0% of all cerebrovascular malformations. The remaining malformations were CAs (two cases, with an incidence of 2.6% in the study population), and DVAs (one case, with an incidence of 1.3% in the study population).

This study has potential limitations. First, the sample size is small, and many gene variants are presented only in single patients. This certainly hinders the possibility to evaluate whether an association exists between these variants and specific cerebrovascular malformations. Additionally, it is known that the rupture of cerebrovascular malformations is devastating in the HHT pediatric population [17,18]. Since our study only includes adult individuals, it might be limited by a survival bias. Additionally, we have been able to analyze only those patients with genetically confirmed HHT who had undergone MRA. Therefore, our sample is not representative of the general HHT population. In addition, since the gold standard for the diagnosis of arteriovenous shunts is catheter angiography and we only had access to MRA data, the incidence of AVFs and microscopic AVMs might be underestimated.

In summary, this study provides updated information on the incidence and distribution of cerebrovascular malformations according to specific gene variants in subjects with HHT. Further studies are needed to substantiate these findings and potentially lead to personalization of risk stratification and screening regimens for cerebrovascular malformations in HHT patients.

Author Contributions: Conceptualization, E.P., F.A., R.P.; methodology, E.G., L.D.M., A.P. (Angelo Porfidia); formal analysis, E.G., E.P., R.P.; investigation, E.G., E.P., F.A., L.D.M., E.L.C., C.L.S., A.P. (Alfredo Puca), A.P. (Angelo Porfidia), A.A., A.P. (Alessandro Pedicelli), R.P.; data curation, E.P., L.D.M., F.A..; writing—original draft preparation, E.G., E.P., R.P.; writing—review and editing, E.G., L.D.M., A.A., R.P.; supervision, E.G., R.P.; project administration, E.G. All authors have read and agreed to the published version of the manuscript.

Funding: This research received no external funding.

Institutional Review Board Statement: This study was conducted in accordance with the Declaration of Helsinki and approved by the Ethics Committee of the Fondazione Policlinico Universitario A. Gemelli IRCCS (protocol number 6241/20, ID 2999, date of approval 20 February 2020).

Informed Consent Statement: Due to the retrospective nature of the study, and the fact that the study only consisted in analysis of data available in the electronic database of our hospital, informed consent was not required.

Data Availability Statement: Data are available upon request to the corresponding author.

Conflicts of Interest: The authors declare no conflict of interest.

References

1. Faughnan, M.E.; Mager, J.J.; Hetts, S.W.; Palda, V.A.; Lang-Robertson, K.; Buscarini, E.; Deslandres, E.; Kasthuri, R.S.; Lausman, A.; Poetker, D.; et al. Second International Guidelines for the Diagnosis and Management of Hereditary Hemorrhagic Telangiectasia. *Ann. Intern. Med.* **2020**, *173*, 989–1001. [CrossRef] [PubMed]
2. Shovlin, C.L.; Buscarini, E.; Kjeldsen, A.D.; Mager, H.J.; Sabba, C.; Droege, F.; Geisthoff, U.; Ugolini, S.; Dupuis-Girod, S. European Reference Network For Rare Vascular Diseases (VASCERN) Outcome Measures For Hereditary Haemorrhagic Telangiectasia (HHT). *Orphanet J. Rare Dis.* **2018**, *13*, 136. [CrossRef] [PubMed]
3. McDonald, J.; Bayrak-Toydemir, P.; Pyeritz, R.E. Hereditary hemorrhagic telangiectasia: An overview of diagnosis, management, and pathogenesis. *Genet. Med.* **2011**, *13*, 607–616. [CrossRef] [PubMed]
4. McAllister, K.A.; Grogg, K.M.; Johnson, D.W.; Gallione, C.J.; Baldwin, M.A.; Jackson, C.E.; Helmbold, E.A.; Markel, D.S.; McKinnon, W.C.; Murrell, J.; et al. Endoglin, a TGF-beta binding protein of endothelial cells, is the gene for hereditary haemorrhagic telangiectasia type 1. *Nat. Genet.* **1994**, *8*, 345. [CrossRef] [PubMed]
5. Johnson, D.W.; Berg, J.N.; Baldwin, M.A.; Gallione, C.J.; Marondel, I.; Yoon, S.J.; Stenzel, T.T.; Speer, M.; Pericak-Vance, M.A.; Diamond, A.; et al. Mutations in the activin receptor-like kinase 1 gene in hereditary haemorrhagic telangiectasia type 2. *Nat. Genet.* **1996**, *13*, 189. [CrossRef] [PubMed]
6. McDonald, J.; Wooderchak-Donahue, W.; VanSant Webb, C.; Whitehead, K.; Stevenson, D.A.; Bayrak-Toydemir, P. Hereditary hemorrhagic telangiectasia: Genetics and molecular diagnostics in a new era. *Front. Genet.* **2015**, *6*, 1. [CrossRef]
7. Gallione, C.J.; Repetto, G.M.; Legius, E.; Rustgi, A.K.; Schelley, S.L.; Tejpar, S.; Mitchell, G.; Drouin, É.; Westermann, C.J.; Marchuk, D.A. A combined syndrome of juvenile polyposis and hereditary haemorrhagic telangiectasia associated with mutations in MADH4 (SMAD4). *Lancet* **2004**, *363*, 852–859. [CrossRef]
8. Albiñana, V.; Zafra, M.P.; Colau, J.; Zarrabeitia, R.; Recio-Poveda, L.; Olavarrieta, L.; Pérez-Pérez, J.; Botella, L.M. Mutation affecting the proximal promoter of Endoglin as the origin of hereditary hemorrhagic telangiectasia type 1. *BMC Med. Genet.* **2017**, *18*, 20. [CrossRef]
9. Sánchez-Martínez, R.; Iriarte, A.; Mora-Luján, J.M.; Patier, J.L.; López-Wolf, D.; Ojeda, A.; Torralba, M.A.; Juyol, M.C.; Gil, R.; Anon, S.; et al. RiHHTa Investigators of the Rare Disease Working Group from the Spanish Society of Internal Medicine. Current HHT Genetic Overview in Spain and its phenotypic Correlation: Data from RiHHTa registry. *Orphanet J. Rare Dis.* **2020**, *15*, 138. [CrossRef]
10. Available online: http://arup.utah.edu/database/ENG/ENG_welcome.php (accessed on 7 March 2022).
11. Woodall, M.N.; McGettigan, M.; Figueroa, R.; Gossage, J.R.; Alleyne, C.H., Jr. Cerebral vascular manifestations in hereditary hemorrhagic telangiectasia. *J. Neurosurg.* **2014**, *120*, 87–92. [CrossRef]
12. Krings, T.; Kim, H.; Power, S.; Nelson, J.; Faughnan, M.E.; Young, W.L.; terBrugge, K.G.; THE Brain Vascular Malformations HHT Investigation Group. Neurovascular Manifestation in Hereditary Hemorrhagic Telangiectasia: Imaging Features and Genotype-Phenotype Correlations. *AJNR Am. J. Neuroradiol.* **2015**, *36*, 863–870. [CrossRef] [PubMed]
13. Brinjikji, W.; Iyer, V.N.; Wood, C.P.; Lanzino, G. Prevalence and characteristics of brain arteriovenous malformations in hereditary hemorrhagic telangiectasia: A systematic review and meta-analysis. *J. Neurosurg.* **2017**, *127*, 302–310. [CrossRef] [PubMed]
14. Brinjikji, W.; Iyer, V.N.; Yamaki, V.; Lanzino, G.; Cloft, H.J.; Thielen, K.R.; Swanson, K.L.; Wood, C.P. Neurovascular Manifestations of Hereditary Hemorrhagic Telangiectasia: A Consecutive Series of 376 Patients during 15 Years. *Am. J. Neuroradiol.* **2016**, *37*, 1479–1486. [CrossRef] [PubMed]
15. Maher, C.O.; Piepgras, D.G.; Brown, D., Jr.; Friedman, J.A.; Pollock, B.E. Cerebrovascular malformations in 321 cases of Hereditary Hemorrhagic Telangiectasia. *Stroke* **2001**, *32*, 877–882. [CrossRef]
16. Ring, N.Y.; Latif, M.A.; Hafezi-Nejad, N.; Holly, B.P.; Weiss, C.R. Prevalence of and Factors Associated with Arterial Aneurysms in Patients with Hereditary Hemorrhagic Telangiectasia: 17-Year Retrospective Series of 418 Patients. *J. Vasc. Interv. Radiol.* **2021**, *32*, 1661–1669. [CrossRef]
17. Morgan, T.; McDonald, J.; Anderson, C.; Ismail, M.; Miller, F.; Mao, R.; Madan, A.; Barnes, P.; Hudgins, L.; Manning, M. Intracranial hemorrhage in infants and children with hereditary hemorrhagic telangiectasia (Osler-Weber-Rendu syndrome). *Pediatrics* **2002**, *109*, e12. [CrossRef]
18. Kilian, A.; Latino, G.A.; White, A.J.; Clark, D.; Chakinala, M.M.; Ratjen, F.; McDonald, J.; Whitehead, K.; Gossage, J.R.; the Brain Vascular Malformation Consortium HHT Investigator Group; et al. Genotype-phenotyipe Correlations in Children with HHT. *J. Clin. Med.* **2020**, *9*, 2714. [CrossRef] [PubMed]

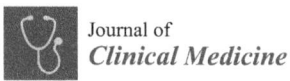

Article

HHT-Related Epistaxis and Pregnancy—A Retrospective Survey and Recommendations for Management from an Otorhinolaryngology Perspective

Kornelia E. C. Andorfer *, Caroline T. Seebauer, Carolin Dienemann, Steven C. Marcrum, René Fischer, Christopher Bohr and Thomas S. Kühnel

Department of Otorhinolaryngology, Regensburg University Medical Center, Franz-Josef-Strauß-Allee 11, 93053 Regensburg, Germany; caroline.seebauer@ukr.de (C.T.S.); carolin.dienemann@stud.uni-regensburg.de (C.D.); steven.marcrum@ukr.de (S.C.M.); rene.fischer@ukr.de (R.F.); christopher.bohr@ukr.de (C.B.); thomas.kuehnel@ukr.de (T.S.K.)
* Correspondence: kornelia.andorfer@ukr.de

Abstract: Appropriate management of hereditary hemorrhagic telangiectasia (HHT) is of particular importance in females, as HHT-mediated modifications of the vascular bed and circulation are known to increase the risk of complications during pregnancy and delivery. This study was undertaken to evaluate female HHT patients' awareness of and experience with HHT during pregnancy and delivery, with a focus on epistaxis. In this retrospective study, 46 females (median age: 60 years) with confirmed HHT completed a 17-item questionnaire assessing knowledge of HHT and its pregnancy-associated complications, the severity of epistaxis during past pregnancies and deliveries, and the desire for better education and counselling regarding HHT and pregnancy. Results revealed that 85% of participants were unaware of their disease status prior to the completion of all pregnancies. Further, 91% reported no knowledge of increased pregnancy-related risk due to HHT. In regard to epistaxis, 61% of respondents reported experiencing nosebleeds during pregnancy. Finally, approximately a third of respondents suggested that receiving counseling on the risks of HHT in pregnancy could have been helpful. Findings suggest that awareness of HHT and its potential for increasing pregnancy-related risk is poor. Best practices in HHT management should be followed to minimize negative effects of the disorder.

Keywords: hereditary hemorrhagic telangiectasia; Morbus Osler; Rendu–Osler–Weber syndrome; Osler Calendar; orphan disease; pregnancy; epistaxis; arteriovenous malformations; laser therapy

Citation: Andorfer, K.E.C.; Seebauer, C.T.; Dienemann, C.; Marcrum, S.C.; Fischer, R.; Bohr, C.; Kühnel, T.S. HHT-Related Epistaxis and Pregnancy—A Retrospective Survey and Recommendations for Management from an Otorhinolaryngology Perspective. *J. Clin. Med.* 2022, 11, 2178. https://doi.org/10.3390/jcm11082178

Academic Editors: Süleyman Ergün and Angel M. Cuesta

Received: 24 February 2022
Accepted: 11 April 2022
Published: 13 April 2022

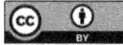

Copyright: © 2022 by the authors. Licensee MDPI, Basel, Switzerland. This article is an open access article distributed under the terms and conditions of the Creative Commons Attribution (CC BY) license (https://creativecommons.org/licenses/by/4.0/).

1. Introduction

Hereditary hemorrhagic telangiectasia (HHT), or Osler–Weber–Rendu disease, is a rare (1:5000) autosomal dominant disorder in which pathological enlargement of blood vessels results in arteriovenous malformations [1]. While any organ can be affected, involvement of the nasal mucosa, skin, lung, gastrointestinal tract, liver and brain are most common [2]. Consensus diagnostic criteria for HHT, known as the Curaçao Criteria, were defined in the year 2000 and include epistaxis, telangiectasias, visceral lesions, and affected first-degree relatives [3].

Epistaxis is the most common manifestation of HHT, which frequently results in diagnosis and management of the disorder being guided by otorhinolaryngologists. Epistaxis due to HHT commonly first presents in puberty [4,5]. However, due to a lack of awareness regarding this rare condition and the fact that symptoms tend to emerge gradually, definitive diagnosis is often first established later in life. For example, Latino et al. reported results of a web-based study in which approximately 40% of respondents described having had consulted an ear, nose and throat (ENT) physician for their epistaxis. On average, however, final diagnosis of HHT did not occur until 14 years after the initial visit [6]. Similarly, Pierucci et al., reported a mean delay in definitive diagnosis exceeding 2 decades, resulting in an average age at diagnosis of approximately 40 years. As a result of delays in recognizing HHT, most patients have completed family planning by the time of diagnosis [7].

In a review of 1577 pregnancies in patients with HHT, Dupuis et al., 2020 reported the incidence of HHT-associated complications during pregnancy to range between 2.7% and 6.8% [8]. Complications related to pulmonary arteriovenous malformations (PAVMs) were most common, comprising a total of 43 events and including hemothorax, hemoptysis, severe hypoxemia and paradoxical emboli with ischemic cerebral stroke and brain abscess. Complications related to hepatic vascular malformations (liver VMs) and cerebral vascular malformations (CVMs) were comparatively rare, though their occurrence could result in similarly serious complications, such as heart failure, hepatobiliary necrosis, or intracranial and spinal bleeding.

Complications during pregnancy are believed to be mediated by hormonal changes, especially during the second and third trimester. For example, modulation of hormone levels has been shown to result in systemic vasodilation, reduced peripheral vascular resistance and an up to 50% increase in cardiac output, with these mechanisms combining to potentially exacerbate blood shunting through preexisting, vulnerable vascular beds [9]. Of particular importance in HHT patients, progesterone-mediated hyperemia and edema of the nasal mucosa have additionally been related to increased frequency and severity of epistaxis. Fortunately, the majority of pregnancies in females with HHT proceed uneventfully. However, when complications do occur, they can be severe and life-threatening for both the mother and child [8,10]. Therefore, screening for and, if indicated, treatment of PAVMs in all females with HHT considering pregnancy should be a priority [10]. Unfortunately, despite the potential exacerbation of epistaxis which may occur during pregnancy due to HHT, recommendations for the management of epistaxis before and during pregnancy are largely missing from the literature.

This study was undertaken to evaluate female HHT patients' understanding of HHT and its potential for increasing pregnancy risks, as well as to characterize their experiences with HHT during pregnancy and delivery, especially as it pertains to epistaxis. The findings were the impetus to deliver recommendations for management of HHT in pregnant women from an otorhinolaryngology perspective and with a focus on epistaxis.

2. Materials and Methods

Fifty-five adult female patients, diagnosed with HHT, were recruited from the outpatient clinic of the Department of Otorhinolaryngology at the University Hospital Regensburg for this retrospective, questionnaire-based study. Inclusion criteria included a definitive diagnosis of HHT, as determined by the presence of at least 3 of 4 Curaçao criteria. Due to the fact that some of the participants had been diagnosed with HHT prior to publication of the Curaçao criteria in the year 2000 or had received their diagnoses external to our clinic, we independently confirmed all HHT diagnoses according to the currently accepted criteria as part of routine follow-up appointments within our day clinic. All participants had a history of at least 1 completed pregnancy and had undergone treatment for nasal telangiectasias in our tertiary referral center between 2019 and 2020. Participants were identified via review of clinical records and were initially contacted by telephone to inform them of the study. Two weeks later, they received a study packet containing additional informing regarding the study, an informed consent form and the 17-item questionnaire (see Appendix A for an English translation). The anonymous questionnaire and the informed consent form were sent back to the study center in 2 separate envelopes, thereby preventing association of questionnaire results with any given respondent. Completed questionnaires and informed consent forms were returned by 46 of the 55 potential respondents. Results from these participants were included in the study and formed the basis of all analyses. All study-related activities were approved by the institutional review board of the University of Regensburg on 13 May 2020 (file number 20-1844-101).

The 17-item questionnaire was divided into four sections: general pregnancy history, awareness of the disease, screening, and treatment of epistaxis. The survey was used to query both the severity of the disease before and during pregnancy, as well as the level of respondent knowledge concerning possible complications. Further, it was intended to assess how females with HHT experienced the disease during pregnancy, especially in terms of epistaxis. Data processing and analysis were performed using SPSS Statistics 25 (International Business Machines Corporation; Armonk, NY, USA). Results were evaluated using descriptive statistics, as appropriate.

3. Results

3.1. General Pregnancy History

Forty-six out of fifty-five (84%) potential respondents returned the questionnaire assessing their personal experiences with HHT and pregnancy and were included in the study. Respondents' ages, provided by 45 out of 46 participants, ranged from 37 to 82 years, with a mean age of 61.7 years (standard deviation (SD) = 11.2 years) at the time of the study. On average, the respondents reported 2.3 pregnancies (SD = 1.6 pregnancies; range = 9 pregnancies) each, resulting in a total of 108 births. Mean age at time of delivery was 27.1 years (SD = 5.3 years; range = 22 years). Two-thirds of the participants provided information on the type of delivery. Briefly, out of 77 deliveries described, vaginal delivery without epidural anesthesia was reported in 61 deliveries (75%), whereas vaginal delivery with epidural anesthesia was reported in 12 deliveries (15%). Finally, cesarean delivery under general anesthesia or epidural anesthesia was performed in four women each (5%).

3.2. Awareness of the Disease

Approximately 84% percent of respondents reported having been diagnosed with HHT only after all pregnancies had been completed (Table 1). Four percent reported receiving the diagnosis after the first, but prior to the last, pregnancy and 11% reported receiving the diagnosis before the first pregnancy. Of significant clinical importance, of the 7 respondents reporting having received the diagnosis prior to the completion of their last pregnancy, 2 stated that having received the HHT diagnosis had influenced their family planning.

Table 1. Timing of HHT diagnosis relative to pregnancy ($n = 45$).

	All Respondents $n = 45$	Age at Survey < 60 Years	Age at Survey > 60 Years
Prior to first pregnancy	5 (11.1%)	3 (13.6%)	2 (8.6%)
Between first and last pregnancy	2 (4.4%)	1 (4.5%)	1 (4.3%)
After last pregnancy	38 (84.4%)	18 (81.8%)	20 (86.9%)

It is possible that diagnostic and counselling procedures have improved over time, such that younger respondents and those with more recent pregnancies might be more likely to report having been informed of their HHT diagnosis prior to the completion of all pregnancies. Results obtained after dividing the respondents into an older and younger group at the arbitrary age of 60 years, the median age of respondents for the dataset, do not suggest a meaningful effect of age on the timepoint of HHT diagnosis (see Table 1). Figures 1 and 2 present dot plots indicating the reported time points of HHT diagnosis as a function of respondent age (Figure 1) and the number of years since the most recent pregnancy (Figure 2). Again, no trend is observable suggesting that younger respondents or more recent mothers are more likely to have received a HHT diagnosis prior to the completion of all pregnancies.

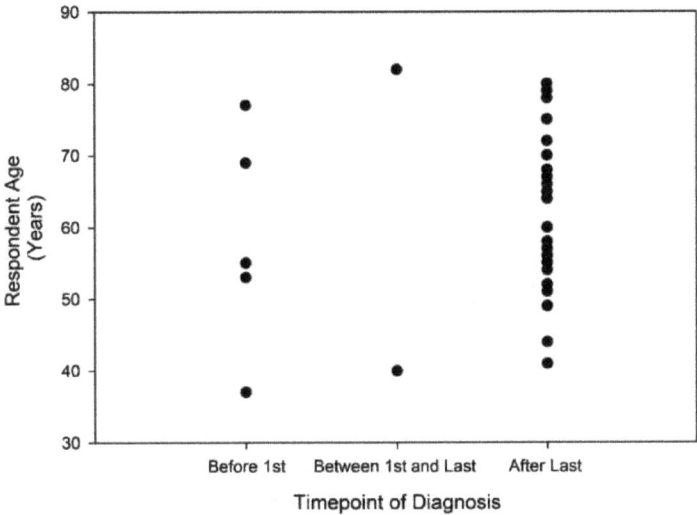

Figure 1. Respondent age as a function of the timepoint of HHT diagnosis.

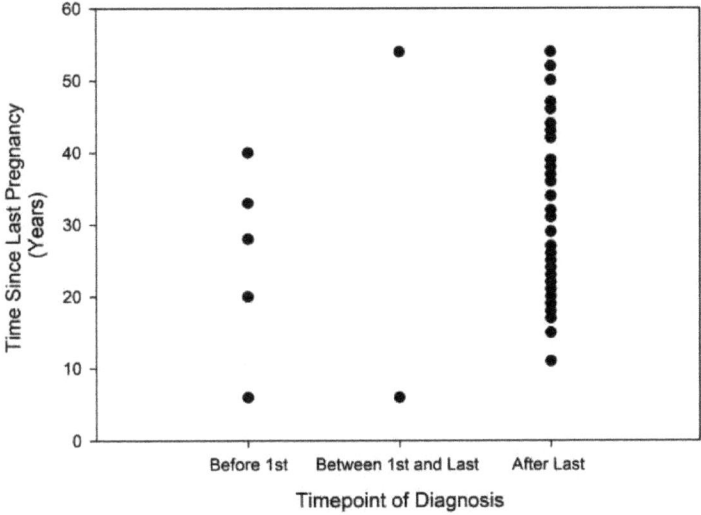

Figure 2. Time since last pregnancy (years) as a function of the timepoint of HHT diagnosis.

3.3. Patient Knowledge and Awareness

At the time of the survey, 42 of 46 respondents (91.3%) reported being generally unaware that HHT is linked to potential complications during pregnancy, while 4 women (8.8%) reported being aware of potential complications. Of these, 2 reported learning of the risks prior to their second pregnancies and 2 learned of the risks after completion of all pregnancies. No respondent reported having had knowledge of the potential risks HHT holds for expectant mothers before onset of the first pregnancy. For respondents younger than 60 years of age, 3 of 22 reported knowing that HHT was associated with complications in pregnancy, while 19 were not aware of any possible disease-related complications. Of the 23 respondents older than 60 years, only one reported knowing about possible complications, while 22 reported not being aware of them. When asked who informed them of potential complications, family members and the treating gynecologist were listed. No respondent reported having been informed about potential complications by an otorhinolaryngologist.

3.4. Screening

Of the 46 total respondents, only 1 reported having received screening for the presence of PAVMs before her pregnancy. Accordingly, 98% of the female HHT patients surveyed did not receive any pre-pregnancy screening. One respondent indicated that she had received treatment to avoid complications due to nose bleeding. In this patient, a skin graft of the thigh was inserted into the nose (septal dermoplasty) to prevent nosebleeds during pregnancy and delivery.

Subgroup analysis revealed that, in the younger age group (younger than 60 years), only one out of 22 responders (4.5%) had received a further examination to clarify organ manifestations associated with HHT. In the older age group, no patient reported further examinations.

3.5. Epistaxis and Treatment

Of the 46 patients who completed the survey, 28 (61%) reported suffering from nosebleeds during their pregnancies. Of these, 46% stated that the severity of the nosebleeds was similar to that of those prior to pregnancy, whereas 27% of respondents reported increased frequency and severity of epistaxis and 27% reported decreased frequency and severity of epistaxis during pregnancy.

Eight of the 28 (29%) respondents affected by epistaxis during pregnancy sought out treatment during pregnancy, while the remaining majority (71%) reported not having needed treatment during pregnancy. For those having received medical treatment for epistaxis, treatment strategies included nasal packing, bipolar cautery, laser therapy and a combination of these measures. When asked whether they were able to self-treat their nasal bleeding, nearly three-quarters of those affected (20 of 28 respondents) answered "yes", one woman (4%) answered with "no" and seven women (25%) said that there was no need for self-treatment at that time. Nasal packing, nasal cooling and nasal ointment were listed as strategies used for self-treatment, when required. Most respondents (91%) reported not experiencing epistaxis during delivery, while 2% of respondents did report nosebleeds and 7% could no longer remember. No participant reported nasal packing as having been necessary during delivery.

Forty-three out of 46 participants answered a subset of questions addressing their desire and need for medical advice and counseling. Thirty-three percent of respondents reported that they would have found professional HHT counseling helpful, 30% said that counseling would not have been helpful and 37% answered the question with "I don't know". Of the 33% (14 participants) who would have found counselling helpful, 9 (64%) suffered from epistaxis during pregnancy, while the remaining 5 participants (36%) had not.

4. Discussion

4.1. Knowledge of Women with HHT about the Disease and Its Complications

A systematic inquiry into diagnostic time delay has suggested that patients receive a definitive diagnosis of HHT more than two decades after the onset of HHT-specific symptoms, on average [7]. Accordingly, family planning is often complete by the time of diagnosis. This finding is in accordance with the results of the retrospective cohort study presented here. We surveyed a total of 46 mothers with HHT who were treated for the disorder in our tertiary referral hospital specialized in the management of HHT. Taken together, over 84% of all respondents indicated that they had received diagnosis of HHT after family planning had been completed. In the majority of cases, pregnancy in females with HHT proceeds uneventfully. In the rare cases in which complications do occur, however, knowledge regarding the disease and its potential effects can play a major role.

A study by Shovlin et al. analyzing 262 pregnancies in 111 women with HHT showed that, in women experiencing a life-threatening event, prior awareness of HHT or PAVM diagnosis was associated with improved survival. In this cohort, the proportion of women not having received the diagnosis of HHT at the time of pregnancy was 74% [10].

In a descriptive case series of 244 pregnancies from Gussem et al., major complications were identified for 13% of women, none of whom had been screened or treated for PAVMs and CVMs prior to pregnancy. In our study, 42 women (91%) indicated that they were not aware of HHT being associated with complications during pregnancy either at the time of pregnancy or at the time of questioning. While international guidelines addressing this topic were recently published, the information does not yet appear to have become common knowledge among female HHT patients. It remains to be seen whether patient age significantly influences knowledge of HHT and pregnancy-related risk, though results of the present study suggest that it might not. None of the remaining four women (9%) who knew about the potential for complications during pregnancy received information before or during their first pregnancy. One patient (2%) was screened for PAVMs prior to the onset of her second pregnancy and another patient (2%) reported having received operative treatment (Saunders operation) to prevent nasal bleeding in preparation for pregnancy.

4.2. Epistaxis during Pregnancy and Delivery in HHT Patients

The results of this study confirm previous reports suggesting both that epistaxis in HHT pregnancies is an important issue for those affected and that there was a general lack of education opportunities and assistance for women with HHT. Nearly two-thirds of the respondents (28/46, 61%) reported having suffered from epistaxis during their pregnancies. The vast majority (85%), however, did not know about their underlying condition at that time. Unfortunately, this is not surprising given the dearth of literature on this topic. In a large retrospective case series, 30.8% of patients reported that they had an increased frequency of epistaxis during pregnancy [11]. This finding is in line with the 27% of respondents reporting increased epistaxis frequency in our survey. To the best of our knowledge, this study is the first to evaluate the course of epistaxis in HHT pregnancies, as neither the recommendations for the management of HHT pregnancies listed in the publication by Shovlin et al., nor the current guidelines, address this issue [10,12].

In our survey, 8 (29%) of 28 respondents stated that their nosebleeds were so pronounced that they needed medical treatment, with treatment strategies including bipolar cautery and laser therapy, nasal packing as well as moisturizing and cooling of the nose. Within the scarce available literature on epistaxis in pregnant women, conservative treatments, such as intravenous tranexamic acid administration, nasal packing and bipolar cautery, are generally recommended as first-line measures. If conservative measures fail, surgical care under general anesthesia may need to be considered [13,14]. The question remains, however, whether these recommendations are generalizable to expectant mothers with HHT.

4.3. Recommendations for Management of Females with HHT from an Otorhinolaryngology Perspective

Results of our survey confirm that there is a need for increased education and counseling efforts on the topic of HHT. Our intention was therefore to provide patients and treating physicians with a clear and short recommendation that could serve as a guide for the management of females with HHT before and during pregnancy. Considerations taken into account in preparation of the presented recommendations summarize information from the current guidelines and literature and are supplemented by us with information on the subject of epistaxis (see Figure 3). For further information on the subject of HHT and pregnancy in general, we highly recommend the current guidelines, which deal with HHT and pregnancy in detail [12].

	prior to pregnancy:	during pregnancy:

ENT	• Instruction for
	  - nasal mucosal care
	  - nasal occlusion
	  - nasal self-packing
	• Coagulation of nasal mucosal lesions with laser and bipolar radiofrequency
	• Planning procedure frequency during pregnancy
		• Repeated instruction for nasal self-packing and prescribing nasal packings
		• Coagulation of nasal mucosal lesions with laser and bipolar radiofrequency under local anaesthesia (Lidocaine topically/ Articaine submucosally)

Interdisciplinary management	• Screening for organ manifestations (pAVMs/cerebral AVMs) • Counselling on rare pregnancy-associated risks	• In the rare case of life-threatening epistaxis, surgical treatment under general anesthesia • Counselling on rare „red-flag" signs indicating pregnancy-associated risks (hemoptysis/ dyspnea) and need for immediate hospitalization if any
Gynecology	• Recommendation for multidisciplinary care in a tertiary center in the presence of untreated PAVMs and/or brainVMs or in the absence of screening for PAVMs • Offer of consultation with a clinical geneticist (for information about family planning, inheritance, penetrance or postnatal genetic testing) • Birth planning taking into account the known visceral manifestations, the family history and the individual medical history of the patient • Completion of the screening measures during pregnancy in accordance with guidelines • Antibiotic prophylaxis during delivery	

Figure 3. Recommendations for Management of HHT-related Epistaxis and Pregnancy from an Otorhinolaryngology Perspective. Items "Interdisciplinary management" and "Gynecology" in keeping with general advice with [10,12]. ENT = Ear, nose and throat physician; HHT = Hereditary hemorrhagic telangiectasia.

The treatment of nasal HHT lesions can be divided into two categories: prevention and therapy. Special attention should be paid to bleeding prevention to avoid the stressful situation of acute, insatiable epistaxis, as well as the potential adverse effects of medication and general anesthesia for the expectant mothers.

As reinforced by our study participants, lubrication of the nasal mucosa with ointment, oils and saline is an established part of basic nasal care and has a preventive effect on nasal bleeding [15]. In addition, we recommend temporal nasal occlusion (tNO) by tape, producing a moist chamber and preventing nasal airflow [16]. Thanks to its simplicity and minimal adverse effects, we consider it convenient as a preventive measure in pregnant women with HHT.

Another key element of prevention is laser treatment, which can be used to treat telangiectasias intranasally with great precision and minimal side effects for the surrounding mucosa [17]. Due to the chronic nature of the disease, laser therapy must be repeated on a regular basis and should, especially during pregnancy, be performed under local anesthesia. We recommend a Blue light laser (445 nm) technique, which is highly specific to blood vessels and HHT lesions, but also Nd:YAG laser or KTP laser treatment is considered suitable [15,17].

As recommended for local anesthetics during pregnancy in dental medicine, we recommend the application of lidocaine topically and articaine submucosally to anesthetize the nasal mucosa prior to treatment [18].

In order to minimize the need for emergency treatment of epistaxis in late-stage pregnancy, at delivery and in the first weeks postpartum, preventive laser treatments are recommended in the months prior to delivery. The frequency of the procedures can be based on the course of complaints documented in an "Osler-Calendar", a tool we created for otorhinolaryngology specialists to review treatment strategies and for patients to enhance their comprehension of the disorder [19].

Bleeding telangiectasias can be treated with high-frequency alternating current, that is, bipolar radiofrequency. Again, treatment under local anesthesia is preferable and a detailed description of the procedure can be obtained elsewhere [15].

The efficacy of systemically administered tranexamic acid (TA) in HHT patients suffering from epistaxis has been established [20,21]. Although it is generally considered safe for intravenous administration, even in acute bleeding during pregnancy and during delivery, according to drug and medication information, it is contraindicated in early pregnancy and should only be used in case of vital threat during late pregnancy [22,23]. Furthermore, there are reports of an HHT-related increase in protein levels of coagulation factor VIII, which promotes thrombotic risk in these patients [24]. Therefore, the continuation of the drug cannot be recommended. In individual cases and for acute emergency treatment with TA, personalized risk-benefit considerations are required. A general recommendation for the use of TA in pregnant HHT patients cannot currently be provided given an inadequate evidence base.

Approximately 61% of women responding to our questionnaire reported being affected by epistaxis during pregnancy. Of these, 71% were able to treat themselves with nasal packings. It is generally accepted that the ability of HHT patients to apply nasal packings without assistance significantly improves quality of life. Thus, our tertiary care center considers training patients in this technique an integral part of the comprehensive care provided [25]. Anemia due to prolonged nasal bleeding can lead to severe complications for both infant and mother [26]. Thus, nasal self-packing is of particular importance for pregnant women with HHT. ENT doctors are generally not on hand at the time of delivery, nor are nasal packings suitable for HHT treatment commonly within reach. Therefore, instruction on self-treatment, as well as the provision of suitable medical nasal packing materials, is a critical part of our recommendations.

To prepare patients for the event of acute nosebleeds, we provide a graduated scheme for nasal self-packing. In mild-to-moderate bleeding, we prefer soft, absorbable sponges (e.g., polyurethane or gelatine), whereas extensive bleeding is best treated with pneumatic nasal packings (PNP). It is important that only tamponades made of smooth material, which is atraumatic for the vulnerable mucous membrane (for example, polyurethane or latex), be used.

In our questionnaire, 1 respondent reported having undergone an operation under general anesthesia in preparation for pregnancy (septal dermoplasty). In no instance was treatment under general anesthesia for acute nasal bleeding necessitated. Information in the literature on how often surgical treatment of epistaxis under general anesthesia is needed in pregnant HHT patients is currently lacking. If the bleeding of nasal lesions appears uncontrollable despite all of the above measures, the need for surgical treatment under general anesthesia is to be discussed with the treating gynecologists and anesthesiologists. Shovlin et al. suggested that, in the rare case of treatment under general anesthesia being required, a modified induction regimen with opiates should be used [10].

As a part of multidisciplinary management, counseling regarding the disease and its pregnancy-associated risks should be provided by several disciplines, including gynecology, otorhinolaryngology and internal medicine. The ENT physician has an important role in this constellation, as the HHT patient is seen by the otorhinolaryngologist prior to the onset of pregnancy most frequently. The following points are to be addressed during the interdisciplinary counseling of pregnant women with HHT and are based on existing guidelines and expert recommendations [10,12]: In the context of pregnancy-associated complications, HHT pregnancies are considered "high risk" if the women have untreated pulmonary AVMs or brain VMs or have not been screened. Women should be advised that there are red-flag symptoms, such as hemoptysis and sudden severe dyspnea. When these symptoms occur, immediate hospitalization is obligatory. In the presence of untreated

PAVMs and/or CVMs, or in the absence of screening for PAVMs, multidisciplinary care in a tertiary center is recommended. In addition, presentation to a clinical geneticist should be advised when the following topics are of particular interest: family planning, inheritance and penetrance of HHT, prenatal diagnostic options, and postnatal genetic testing.

Further aspects must be considered in the context of gynecological care. Namely, scheduling of the delivery must account for the known visceral manifestations, the family history and the individual medical history of the patient. Screening for visceral manifestations during pregnancy must be obtained in accordance with guidelines. For all pregnant women with HHT, antibiotic prophylaxis during delivery is recommended [10,12].

4.4. Future Research Directions

The findings of this study are limited in several aspects, each of which represents a direction for future research. First, the relatively long period of time between the participants' pregnancies and the time of the survey increases the probability that participants recalled HHT-related details from past pregnancies inaccurately. Future work assessing the experiences of mothers with HHT more closely following childbirth is needed to better account for recall bias in study results. However, given that most women of childbearing age will not yet have received a reliable HHT diagnosis, the value of retrospective studies with longer intervals should not be underestimated. Further, as the older mothers included in our sample serve as valuable sources of HHT-related information to their children, we consider results describing their experience with and knowledge of HHT to be of significant clinical interest. Second, given the high median age of participants in our sample (60 years), it is possible that their experience is no longer reflective of that of younger mothers with HHT. For example, recent efforts in terms of early diagnosis of HHT and patient education suggest that a younger participant cohort might possess a greater level of knowledge and awareness on the topic than did our older cohort. Such an effect would serve to limit the generalizability of our findings. Importantly, though limited in terms of sample size, this study included respondents as young as 37 years and results did not reveal any effect of participant age. For example, results of our subgroup analysis indicated that reports from participants older than 60 years were similar to those of the younger participants. As such, time since the most recent pregnancy might not be as great a limiting factor as might initially be presumed. Additional studies are needed to systematically assess for any effect of age on a patient's experience with HHT and pregnancy. Third, while difficult to avoid in the context of a single-center trial evaluating a rare disease such as HHT, with only 85,000 HHT patients in Europe, more females than males with different clinical presentations, the small sample size precluded advanced statistical evaluation [27,28]. Longer-term and multi-center study designs should be considered in future work to overcome these limitations and provide much-needed detail in this area.

5. Conclusions

The recommendations for management of HHT in pregnant women from an otorhinolaryngology perspective, formulated as a consequence of our study results, are not intended to replace existing guidelines. Rather, these recommendations are designed to complement available guidelines and help close a gap in knowledge about epistaxis in pregnant women with HHT. Results of the present study indicate a significant need for appropriate counseling on the manifestations of HHT in pregnancy. To achieve this, increased awareness of this disease among health care professionals, in particular ENT doctors and emergency physicians, is critical. However, it is just as important that medical information on HHT be received by affected patients. Women with HHT must be educated about organ screening, medical treatment and self-treatment of epistaxis and possible pregnancy-related complications prior to pregnancy. The knowledge and implementation of recommendations for management of HHT pregnancies is indispensable in reducing the rare but potentially life-threatening complications of HHT during pregnancy.

Author Contributions: K.E.C.A. contributed as a first author and ENT physician by creating the study design, preparing the study, reviewing the literature and writing the manuscript. C.B. and T.S.K. participated in the design of the study. C.D., C.T.S., R.F. and S.C.M. collected data and helped with figures and statistics. S.C.M., C.T.S. and T.S.K. helped to draft the manuscript. All authors have read and agreed to the published version of the manuscript.

Funding: This research received no external funding.

Institutional Review Board Statement: The study was conducted in accordance with the Declaration of Helsinki, and approved by the institutional review board of the University of Regensburg (file number 20-1844-101, date of approval 13 May 2020).

Informed Consent Statement: Informed consent was obtained from all subjects involved in the study.

Data Availability Statement: The datasets used and analyzed during the current study are available from the corresponding author upon reasonable request.

Acknowledgments: The authors very much appreciate the support from Birgit Scheungrab.

Conflicts of Interest: The authors declare no conflict of interest.

Appendix A

1. How many children do you have and how old were you at the time of each delivery?

    Number of children |__|
    Age at delivery:
    First delivery |__|__|
    Second delivery |__|__|
    Third delivery |__|__|
    Please list any additional delivery and your age at the time of delivery here:_____

2. When did you learn that you have HHT?
    - ○ before the onset of my first pregnancy
    - ○ before the onset of pregnancy number |__|
    - ○ during pregnancy number |__|
    - ○ after completion of all pregnancies

3. Has your illness influenced your family planning or desire to have children?
    - ○ no
    - ○ yes

4. Are you currently aware that HHT is linked to an increased likelihood of complications during pregnancy (for example, pulmonary bleeding, heart problems or increased risk of stroke)?
    - ○ no
    - ○ yes

    4.1. If you answered "yes" to Question 4, were you aware before your pregnancy(ies)?
    - ○ no
    - ○ yes
    - ○ I have had multiple pregnancies. I was not aware before the first pregnancy, but was aware before subsequent pregnancy(ies).

5. If you answered either "yes" or "I have had multiple pregnancies." to question 4.1, please answer the following question.

    Who informed you about the possibility of complications during pregnancy (for example, pulmonary bleeding, heart problems or increased risk of stroke)?
    - ○ general/primary care practitioner
    - ○ Ear-Nose-and-Throat doctor
    - ○ family members

○ HHT support group
○ Others: _____

6. Did you have HHT-related examinations of the lungs, liver, brain, spine or gastrointestinal tract prior to or during your pregnancy(ies)?
   ○ no
   ○ yes

   If yes, which examinations (select all that apply)?
   ○ Inspection of the lung (ultrasound/CT scan/pulmonary function test)
   ○ Inspection of the liver (ultrasound)
   ○ Inspection of the brain (MRI)
   ○ Inspection of the spine (MRI)

7. Did you undergo any medical treatments before or during your pregnancy(ies) to reduce the likelihood of HHT-related complications (e.g., embolization of AV shunts of the lung, liver or brain)?
   ○ no
   ○ yes

   If yes, please list the treatments:_____

   For questions 8–14, please provide responses in reference to the pregnancy during which nosebleeds were the most intense and disturbing.

8. Did you have nosebleeds during this pregnancy?
   ○ no
   ○ yes

   If yes, how intense were the nosebleeds compared to before pregnancy?
   ○ more intense
   ○ same intensity
   ○ less intense

9. Did your nosebleeds need to be treated during this pregnancy (more than the external use of a tissue?)?
   ○ no
   ○ yes

   If yes, please tick the method/s used?
   ○ Self-tamponade
   ○ Tamponade via a health care professional
   ○ cautery
   ○ laser treatment
   ○ cautery/laser treatment or embolization under general anesthesia

10. If you answered "yes" to Question 8, would you have been capable of treating your nosebleeds yourself (for example, by self-tamponade)?
    ○ was not necessary
    ○ no
    ○ yes

    If yes, how _____

11. Did you have nosebleeds during delivery?
    ○ no
    ○ yes
    ○ Don't know/cannot remember

12. Did you have to pack your nose during delivery?
    ○ no

- ○ yes
- ○ Don't know/cannot remember

13. We would now like to know how satisfied you were with your nosebleeds during pregnancy.

    Please tick the appropriate number on the subjective, numeric rating scale (NRS).

0	1	2	3	4	5	6	7	8	9	10
○	○	○	○	○	○	○	○	○	○	○

    0 = completely unsatisfied; 10 = completely satisfied.

14. We want to know how satisfied you were with your nosebleeds during delivery.

    Please tick the appropriate number on the subjective, numeric rating scale (NRS).

0	1	2	3	4	5	6	7	8	9	10
○	○	○	○	○	○	○	○	○	○	○

    0 = completely unsatisfied; 10 = completely satisfied.

15. What kind of birth/births did you have? Specify the number:
    - |__| time/s spontaneous delivery with epidural anesthesia
    - |__| time/s spontaneous delivery without epidural anesthesia
    - |__| time/s c-section with epidural anesthesia
    - |__| time/s c-section under general anesthesia

16. Would you have found medical advice on HHT during your pregnancy(ies) helpful?
    - ○ no
    - ○ yes
    - ○ I don't know

17. How old are you now? _____ years

References

1. Dakeishi, M.; Shioya, T.; Wada, Y.; Shindo, T.; Otaka, K.; Manabe, M.; Nozaki, J.-I.; Inoue, S.; Koizumi, A. Genetic epidemiology of hereditary hemorrhagic telangiectasia in a local community in the northern part of Japan. *Hum. Mutat.* **2002**, *19*, 140–148. [CrossRef] [PubMed]
2. Faughnan, M.E.; Palda, V.A.; Garcia-Tsao, G.; Geisthoff, U.W.; McDonald, J.; Proctor, D.D.; Spears, J.; Brown, D.H.; Buscarini, E.; Chesnutt, M.S.; et al. International guidelines for the diagnosis and management of hereditary haemorrhagic telangiectasia. *J. Med. Genet.* **2011**, *48*, 73–87. [CrossRef] [PubMed]
3. Shovlin, C.L.; Guttmacher, A.E.; Buscarini, E.; Faughnan, M.E.; Hyland, R.H.; Westermann, C.J.; Kjeldsen, A.D.; Plauchu, H. Diagnostic criteria for hereditary hemorrhagic telangiectasia (Rendu-Osler-Weber syndrome). *Am. J. Med Genet.* **2000**, *91*, 66–67. [CrossRef]
4. Plauchu, H.; De Chadarévian, J.-P.; Bideau, A.; Robert, J.-M. Age-related clinical profile of hereditary hemorrhagic telangiectasia in an epidemiologically recruited population. *Am. J. Med. Genet.* **1989**, *32*, 291–297. [CrossRef] [PubMed]
5. Assar, O.S.; Friedman, C.M.; White, R.I.J. The natural history of epistaxis in hereditary hemorrhagic telangiectasia. *Laryngoscope.* **1991**, *101*, 977–980. [CrossRef]
6. Latino, G.A.; Brown, D.; Glazier, R.H.; Weyman, J.T.; Faughnan, M.E. Targeting under-diagnosis in hereditary hemorrhagic telangiectasia: A model approach for rare diseases? *Orphanet J. Rare Dis.* **2014**, *9*, 115. [CrossRef]
7. Pierucci, P.; Lenato, G.M.; Suppressa, P.; Lastella, P.; Triggiani, V.; Valerio, R.; Comelli, M.; Salvante, D.; Stella, A.; Resta, N.; et al. A long diagnostic delay in patients with Hereditary Haemorrhagic Telangiectasia: A questionnaire-based retrospective study. *Orphanet J. Rare Dis.* **2012**, *7*, 33. [CrossRef]
8. Dupuis, O.; Delagrange, L.; Dupuis-Girod, S. Hereditary haemorrhagic telangiectasia and pregnancy: A review of the literature. *Orphanet J. Rare Dis.* **2020**, *15*, 5. [CrossRef]
9. Silversides, C.K.; Colman, J.M. Physiological Changes in Pregnancy. In *Heart Disease in Pregnancy*; John Wiley & Sons, Ltd.: Hoboken, NJ, USA, 2007; pp. 6–17. [CrossRef]
10. Shovlin, C.L.; Sodhi, V.; McCarthy, A.; Lasjaunias, P.; Jackson, J.E.; Sheppard, M.N. Estimates of maternal risks of pregnancy for women with hereditary haemorrhagic telangiectasia (Osler-Weber-Rendu syndrome): Suggested approach for obstetric services. *BJOG* **2008**, *115*, 1108–1115. [CrossRef]
11. de Gussem, E.M.; Lausman, A.Y.; Beder, A.J.; Edwards, C.P.; Blanker, M.H.; Terbrugge, K.G.; Mager, J.J.; Faughnan, M.E. Outcomes of pregnancy in women with hereditary hemorrhagic telangiectasia. *Obstet. Gynecol.* **2014**, *123*, 514–520. [CrossRef]

12. Faughnan, M.E.; Mager, J.J.; Hetts, S.W.; Palda, V.A.; Lang-Robertson, K.; Buscarini, E.; Deslandres, E.; Kasthuri, R.S.; Lausman, A.; Poetker, D.; et al. Second International Guidelines for the Diagnosis and Management of Hereditary Hemorrhagic Telangiectasia. *Ann. Intern. Med.* **2020**, *173*, 989–1001. [CrossRef] [PubMed]
13. Giambanco, L.; Iannone, V.; Borriello, M.; Scibilia, G.; Scollo, P. The way a nose could affect pregnancy: Severe and recurrent epistaxis. *Pan Afr. Med J.* **2019**, *34*, 49. [CrossRef] [PubMed]
14. Piccioni, M.G.; Derme, M.; Salerno, L.; Morrocchi, E.; Pecorini, F.; Porpora, M.G.; Brunelli, R. Management of Severe Epistaxis during Pregnancy: A Case Report and Review of the Literature. *Case Rep. Obstet. Gynecol.* **2019**, *2019*, 5825309. [CrossRef] [PubMed]
15. Wirsching, K.E.C.; Kühnel, T.S. Update on Clinical Strategies in Hereditary Hemorrhagic Telangiectasia from an ENT Point of View. *Clin. Exp. Otorhinolaryngol.* **2017**, *10*, 153–157. [CrossRef] [PubMed]
16. Wirsching, K.E.C.; Haubner, F.; Kühnel, T.S. Influence of temporary nasal occlusion (tNO) on epistaxis frequency in patients with hereditary hemorrhagic telangiectasia (HHT). *Eur. Arch. Oto-Rhino-Laryngol.* **2017**, *274*, 1891–1896. [CrossRef] [PubMed]
17. Bertlich, M.; Kashani, F.; Weiss, B.G.; Wiebringhaus, R.; Ihler, F.; Freytag, S.; Gires, O.; Kühnel, T.; Haubner, F. Safety and Efficacy of Blue Light Laser Treatment in Hereditary Hemorrhagic Telangiectasia. *Lasers Surg. Med.* **2021**, *53*, 309–315. [CrossRef]
18. Ouanounou, A.; Haas, D.A. Drug therapy during pregnancy: Implications for dental practice. *Br. Dent. J.* **2016**, *220*, 413–417. [CrossRef]
19. Seebauer, C.T.; Freigang, V.; Schwan, F.E.; Fischer, R.; Bohr, C.; Kühnel, T.S.; Andorfer, K.E.C. Hereditary Hemorrhagic Telangiectasia: Success of the Osler Calendar for Documentation of Treatment and Course of Disease. *J. Clin. Med.* **2021**, *10*, 4720. [CrossRef]
20. Gaillard, S.; Dupuis-Girod, S.; Boutitie, F.; Rivière, S.; Morinière, S.; Hatron, P.-Y.; Manfredi, G.; Kaminsky, P.; Capitaine, A.-L.; Roy, P.; et al. Tranexamic acid for epistaxis in hereditary telangiectasia patients: A European cross-over controlled trial in a rare disease. *J. Thromb. Haemost.* **2014**, *12*, 1494–1502. [CrossRef]
21. Albiñana, V.; Cuesta, A.M.; De Rojas, P.I.; Gallardo-Vara, E.; Recio-Poveda, L.; Bernabéu, C.; Botella, L.M. Review of Pharmacological Strategies with Repurposed Drugs for Hereditary Telangiectasia Related Bleeding. *J. Clin. Med.* **2020**, *9*, 1766. [CrossRef]
22. Peitsidis, P.; Kadir, R.A. Antifibrinolytic therapy with tranexamic acid in pregnancy and postpartum. *Expert Opin. Pharmacother.* **2011**, *12*, 503–516. [CrossRef] [PubMed]
23. Shakur-Still, H.; Roberts, I.; Fawole, B.; Chaudhri, R.; El-Sheikh, M.; Akintan, A.; Qureshi, Z.; Kidanto, H.; Vwalika, B.; Abdulkadir, A.; et al. Effect of early tranexamic acid administration on mortality, hysterectomy, and other morbidities in women with post-partum haemorrhage (WOMAN): An international, randomised, double-blind, placebo-controlled trial. *Lancet* **2017**, *389*, 2105–2116. [CrossRef]
24. Shovlin, C.L.; Sulaiman, N.L.; Govani, F.S.; Jackson, J.E.; Begbie, M.E. Elevated factor VIII in hereditary haemorrhagic telangiectasia (HHT): Association with venous thromboembolism. *Thromb. Haemost.* **2007**, *98*, 1031–1039.
25. Droege, F.; Lueb, C.; Thangavelu, K.; Stuck, B.A.; Lang, S.; Geisthoff, U. Nasal self-packing for epistaxis in Hereditary Hemorrhagic Telangiectasia increases quality of life. *Rhinology* **2019**, *57*, 231–239. [CrossRef]
26. Williams, M.D.; Wheby, M.S. Anemia in pregnancy. *Med Clin. N. Am.* **1992**, *76*, 631–647. [CrossRef]
27. Shovlin, C.L.; Buscarini, E.; Kjeldsen, A.D.; Mager, H.J.; Sabba, C.; Droege, F.; Geisthoff, U.; Ugolini, S.; Dupuis-Girod, S. European Reference Network for Rare Vascular Diseases (VASCERN) Outcome Measures for Hereditary Haemorrhagic Telangiectasia (HHT). *Orphanet. J. Rare Dis.* **2018**, *13*, 136. [CrossRef]
28. Mora-Luján, J.M.; Iriarte, A.; Alba, E.; Sánchez-Corral, M.A.; Cerdà, P.; Cruellas, F.; Ordi, Q.; Corbella, X.; Ribas, J.; Castellote, J.; et al. Gender differences in hereditary hemorrhagic telangiectasia severity. *Orphanet J. Rare Dis.* **2020**, *15*, 63. [CrossRef]

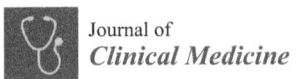

Article

Hereditary Hemorrhagic Telangiectasia: Success of the Osler Calendar for Documentation of Treatment and Course of Disease

Caroline T. Seebauer [1,*], Viola Freigang [2], Franziska E. Schwan [1], René Fischer [1], Christopher Bohr [1], Thomas S. Kühnel [1] and Kornelia E. C. Andorfer [1]

[1] Department of Otorhinolaryngology, Regensburg University Medical Center, Franz-Josef-Strauß-Allee 11, 93053 Regensburg, Germany; franziska.schwan@ukr.de (F.E.S.); rene.fischer@ukr.de (R.F.); christopher.bohr@ukr.de (C.B.); thomas.kuehnel@ukr.de (T.S.K.); kornelia.andorfer@ukr.de (K.E.C.A.)
[2] Department of Trauma, Regensburg University Medical Center, Franz-Josef-Strauß-Allee 11, 93053 Regensburg, Germany; viola.freigang@ukr.de
* Correspondence: caroline.seebauer@ukr.de

Abstract: Hereditary hemorrhagic telangiectasia (HHT; Rendu-Osler-Weber syndrome) affects the capillary and larger vessels, leading to arteriovenous shunts. Epistaxis is the main symptom impairing quality of life. The aim of the Osler Calendar is to offer information about the extent of the systemic disease and the current state of treatment. A care plan with information on the rare disease and self-treatment of epistaxis was created. Organ examinations and ongoing treatments were recorded. A questionnaire documents the treatment success, including patient satisfaction, frequency of hemorrhage and hemoglobin levels. The patients using the Osler Calendar for at least one year ($n = 54$) were surveyed. Eighty-five percent of patients ($n = 46$) used the calendar to gain information about HHT. Seventy-two percent ($n = 39$) used the Osler Calendar for instructions on the self-treatment of nosebleeds. The calendar increased patients' understanding for the need for organ screenings from 48% ($n = 26$) to 81% ($n = 44$). Seventy-nine percent ($n = 43$) of patients confirmed that the Osler Calendar documented their therapeutic process either well or very well. Fifty-two percent ($n = 28$) saw an improvement in the therapeutic process due to the documentation. The Osler Calendar records the individual intensity of the disease and facilitates the communication between attending physicians. It is a tool for specialists to review treatment strategies. Furthermore, the calendar enhances patients' comprehension of their condition.

Keywords: hereditary hemorrhagic telangiectasia; Morbus Osler; Rendu-Osler-Weber syndrome; Osler Calendar; orphan disease; epistaxis; arteriovenous malformations; organ manifestation; screening; laser therapy

Citation: Seebauer, C.T.; Freigang, V.; Schwan, F.E.; Fischer, R.; Bohr, C.; Kühnel, T.S.; Andorfer, K.E.C. Hereditary Hemorrhagic Telangiectasia: Success of the Osler Calendar for Documentation of Treatment and Course of Disease. *J. Clin. Med.* **2021**, *10*, 4720. https://doi.org/10.3390/jcm10204720

Academic Editor: Angel M. Cuesta

Received: 31 August 2021
Accepted: 10 October 2021
Published: 14 October 2021

Publisher's Note: MDPI stays neutral with regard to jurisdictional claims in published maps and institutional affiliations.

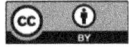

Copyright: © 2021 by the authors. Licensee MDPI, Basel, Switzerland. This article is an open access article distributed under the terms and conditions of the Creative Commons Attribution (CC BY) license (https://creativecommons.org/licenses/by/4.0/).

1. Introduction

Hereditary hemorrhagic telangiectasia (HHT; Rendu-Osler-Weber syndrome) is an autosomal, dominant, inherited disorder affecting the capillary and larger vessels in all organs in the human body. The occurring lesions range from very small microvascular dilatations to arteriovenous shunts with a diameter of several centimeters. These vascular malformations can be predominantly found in the nasal mucosa, intestine, lung, liver and the central nervous system.

HHT occurs with a prevalence of between 1:5000 and 1:8000 [1]. Thus, HHT belongs to a category of orphan diseases and should be treated in specialized centers [2]. However, in everyday life patients are in contact with healthcare providers with limited prior exposure or training on this specific disease [3]. A diagnosis is based on clinical symptoms, referred to as the Curaçao criteria. These criteria comprise epistaxis, visceral lesions, a positive family history and telangiectasias involving the perioral region, tongue, oral mucosa and fingers [2]. If at least three of these four criteria are fulfilled, the diagnosis can be regarded as definite. Where only two criteria are satisfied, HHT is possible or suspected [4]. Without genetical testing a suspected diagnosis cannot be discounted as further symptoms may occur over time. Epistaxis is the main presenting symptom and almost every patient diagnosed with HHT is affected by it. The intensity of this symptom varies from mild, scarce bleeding to life-threatening epistaxis requiring nasal packing, hospitalization, and frequent blood transfusion, thus limiting the patient's quality of life [5]. The current therapeutic strategies follow an algorithm that takes an individualized account of the severity of epistaxis and quality of life [6]. A multistage concept for HHT nose bleeds includes laser therapy and surgery, as well as drug therapies. In addition, screening examinations to determine the effects of the internal organs (mainly lung, liver, brain, and gastro-intestinal tract) are carried out. Visceral lesions which require treatment, should be treated in interdisciplinary cooperation with the corresponding specialized department.

Currently, there is no standardized tool to record treatment success or show the need for the escalation of treatment. With HHT being an orphan disease, patients are aware that the knowledge of non-specialized physicians about HHT is limited. Therefore, information about Rendu-Osler-Weber syndrome, the self-treatment of epistaxis, antibiotic prophylaxis and the necessary organ examinations are crucial for attending physicians and patients. To increase awareness of this rare disease and to document the ongoing treatment by the specialized center, a patient brochure in combination with a treatment documentation tool was developed.

2. Materials and Methods

2.1. Osler Calendar

Being part of the center of orphan diseases at the Regensburg University Medical Center, the Department of Otorhinolaryngology developed a care plan, called the Osler Calendar, for patients with HHT and their attending physicians. The aim was to provide basic knowledge about the disease such as how to self-manage the symptom of acute epistaxis and when antibiotic prophylaxis is necessary. Additionally, the calendar focused on the need of organ screening examination and its documentation. At last, the calendar documented the patient's satisfaction and clinical parameters next to the therapy conducted by the specialized center. For a PDF version of the Osler Calendar see Supplementary Materials.

2.2. Multistep Treatment Approach

From January 2018 onwards, the treatment of HHT patients at the Department of Otorhinolaryngology at the Regensburg University Medical Center was documented with the Osler Calendar. The first step of the multistep treatment approach was protecting the nasal mucosa by daily application of creams, oils, splints, hygroscopic sprays or temporary nasal occlusion with adhesive plaster [7]. The next step comprised the use of pulsed Nd:YAG laser (infrared 1064 nm) and the TruBlue laser (blue light 445 nm) [5,8]. Coagulation with high-frequency alternating current was used on high-flow shunts. If these measures failed to succeed, surgery was indicated to close feeding vessels or the nidus was resected [1]. In some patients, local endonasal administration of 3.75 mg Bevacizumab per side was conducted in addition to laser therapy or surgery [9]. Patients not eligible for surgical intervention or suffering from blood loss due to visceral lesion, received systemic Bevacizumab treatment according to previously published protocols [10].

2.3. Patients

A questionnaire was handed to patients ($n = 54$), who received treatment for HHT at a tertiary referral center specializing in HHT between 2019 and 2020. All patients were diagnosed with HHT clinically according to the Curaçao criteria (all patients were positive for at least three out of four criteria) and used the Osler Calendar for at least one year. Pediatric patients were excluded from this study, as symptoms requiring interventions usually occurred later in life. This retrospective descriptive study was based on an anonymous survey using a questionnaire developed to evaluate the use of the Osler Calendar.

The study was conducted at the Department of Otorhinolaryngology, University Medical Center Regensburg, Germany, according to the principles of Helsinki and approved by the Local Ethics Committee (No. 17-854-101). Informed consent was obtained from all subjects involved in the study.

2.4. Questionnaire to Review the Osler Calendar from the Patient's Point of View

Thirteen months after introducing the Osler Calendar to our clinical routine we evaluated current treatment strategies based on the information given by the Osler-Calendar and reviewed the calendar from the patient's point of view. A questionnaire was developed to determine if patients used the Osler Calendar for information about their disease, self-treatment of epistaxis, antibiotic prophylaxis, and necessary organ screening examinations. Those questions were answered with yes or no. The questions, if organ-screening was important to patients before and after the use of the Osler Calendar and if the Osler Calendar documented the course of the disease adequately, were answered by a five-point likert scale. The questions of whether attending physicians of patients with HHT used the Osler Calendar for information about the disease and the ongoing treatment were answered with yes or no. A three-point likert scale was applied to answer the question of whether the Osler Calendar improved patient's treatment and a visual analogue scale from zero to ten answered how content patients were regarding the frequency of epistaxis.

2.5. Statistics

Data processing and statistical analysis was based on the statistics software, SPSS Statistics 25 (International Business Machines Corporation; Armonk, NY, USA). Microsoft Excel (©2021 Microsoft Corporation) was used for data collection and the displaying of results. Categorical or nominal data were shown in pie charts. The graphs displayed the number of patients in the upper row and the percentage of all patients ($n = 54$) in the lower row. Results of the visual analogue scale were displayed as box plot (medians and interquartile range).

3. Osler Calendar Content and Results

3.1. Information on HHT and Self-Treatment for Nosebleeds

The first aim of the Osler Calendar was to inform patients briefly about the most common symptoms of Osler-Weber-Rendu syndrome and how to approach them (Figure 1A). The most common symptom is epistaxis, which occurs in over 90% of cases. Nosebleeds are caused by vascular malformations which appear in the mucous membranes of the nose, but also in the intestine, lungs, liver, and brain. Currently, the disease is incurable, and the symptoms cannot be permanently alleviated. The main aim of treatment is to lengthen the intervals between bleedings, to reduce the intensity of bleeding, to contain the spread of the disease and to prevent the complications resulting from visceral lesions (see Section 3.2). The treatment of the nasal mucosa follows a multi-step approach, where the first step is the prevention of bleeding thorough the care of the mucous membranes by the patient with a soft nose ointment or nose oil. It can also be helpful to limit nasal breathing temporarily by closing the nostrils with plasters (e.g., Micropore™ 2.5 cm or hydrocolloid nasal tape). Thus the mucous membranes are protected from drying out, crusting and microtrauma due to air flow [7,11,12]. These "second-hits" are discussed in the literature for triggering the growth of the lesions [13]. In acute situations, decongestant nasal gel or spray, compression of the nose, and blood pressure monitoring are recommended. For more severe bleedings, nasal inserts (e.g., Stypro® Standard, Curasan; NasoPore® Standard, Stryker, Kalamazoo, MI, USA), which may be soaked with decongestant nose drops or tranexamic acid (500 mg/5 mL), can be prescribed to the patient. For epistaxis, which is not controlled by these measures, carboxymethyl cellulose nasal dressings (e.g., Rapid Rhino™ Gel-Knit, Smith & Nephew) and inflatable nasal tamponades (e.g., Rapid Rhino™, Smith & Nephew) are available. The Osler Calendar provides an overview of the disease pattern of HHT and provides online links where patients can find more detailed information. After one year of using the Osler Calendar, 85% of patients ($n = 46$) claimed to use the calendar to gain information about Osler-Weber-Rendu disease (Figure 1B, left panel). Furthermore, the Osler Calendar informed patients of how to approach nosebleeds of varying severities and provided detailed instructions on nasal packing. Seventy two percent ($n = 39$) of patients stated, that they used the Osler Calendar for instructions about self-treatment for nosebleed (Figure 1B, right panel).

A

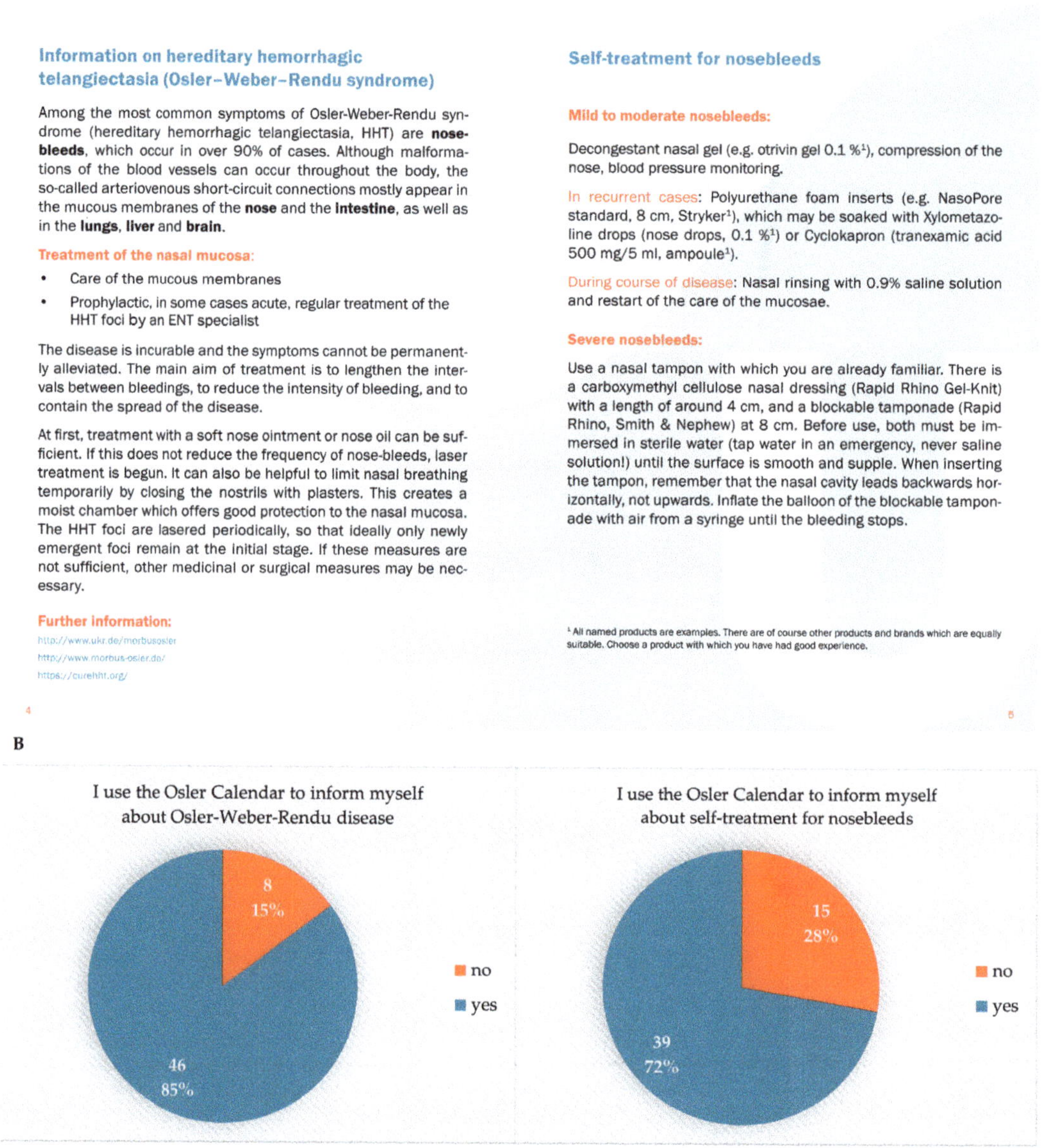

Information on hereditary hemorrhagic telangiectasia (Osler–Weber–Rendu syndrome)

Among the most common symptoms of Osler-Weber-Rendu syndrome (hereditary hemorrhagic telangiectasia, HHT) are **nosebleeds**, which occur in over 90% of cases. Although malformations of the blood vessels can occur throughout the body, the so-called arteriovenous short-circuit connections mostly appear in the mucous membranes of the **nose** and the **intestine**, as well as in the **lungs**, **liver** and **brain**.

Treatment of the nasal mucosa:
- Care of the mucous membranes
- Prophylactic, in some cases acute, regular treatment of the HHT foci by an ENT specialist

The disease is incurable and the symptoms cannot be permanently alleviated. The main aim of treatment is to lengthen the intervals between bleedings, to reduce the intensity of bleeding, and to contain the spread of the disease.

At first, treatment with a soft nose ointment or nose oil can be sufficient. If this does not reduce the frequency of nose-bleeds, laser treatment is begun. It can also be helpful to limit nasal breathing temporarily by closing the nostrils with plasters. This creates a moist chamber which offers good protection to the nasal mucosa. The HHT foci are lasered periodically, so that ideally only newly emergent foci remain at the initial stage. If these measures are not sufficient, other medicinal or surgical measures may be necessary.

Further information:
http://www.ukr.de/morbusosler
http://www.morbus-osler.de/
https://curehht.org/

Self-treatment for nosebleeds

Mild to moderate nosebleeds:

Decongestant nasal gel (e.g. otrivin gel 0.1 %[1]), compression of the nose, blood pressure monitoring.

In recurrent cases: Polyurethane foam inserts (e.g. NasoPore standard, 8 cm, Stryker[1]), which may be soaked with Xylometazoline drops (nose drops, 0.1 %[1]) or Cyclokapron (tranexamic acid 500 mg/5 ml, ampoule[1]).

During course of disease: Nasal rinsing with 0.9% saline solution and restart of the care of the mucosae.

Severe nosebleeds:

Use a nasal tampon with which you are already familiar. There is a carboxymethyl cellulose nasal dressing (Rapid Rhino Gel-Knit) with a length of around 4 cm, and a blockable tamponade (Rapid Rhino, Smith & Nephew) at 8 cm. Before use, both must be immersed in sterile water (tap water in an emergency, never saline solution!) until the surface is smooth and supple. When inserting the tampon, remember that the nasal cavity leads backwards horizontally, not upwards. Inflate the balloon of the blockable tamponade with air from a syringe until the bleeding stops.

[1] All named products are examples. There are of course other products and brands which are equally suitable. Choose a product with which you have had good experience.

B

I use the Osler Calendar to inform myself about Osler-Weber-Rendu disease
- no: 8 (15%)
- yes: 46 (85%)

I use the Osler Calendar to inform myself about self-treatment for nosebleeds
- no: 15 (28%)
- yes: 39 (72%)

Figure 1. (**A**) Information on HHT and self-treatment for nosebleeds. (**B**) Use of the Osler Calendar for information on HHT and self-treatment of nosebleeds.

3.2. Information on Screening Examinations for Visceral Lesions of HHT

According to the Second International Guidelines for the Diagnosis and Management of HHT, screening examinations for visceral lesions are recommended [2]. All patients with possible or confirmed HHT should be screened for vascular anomalies involving the lungs, liver and the brain. The screening for pulmonary arteriovenous malformations (PAVM) is performed by a transthoracic contrast echocardiography as the initial screening test. In case PAVMs are suspected, the diagnosis is confirmed or dismissed by contrast-enhanced, thoracic, computed tomography (CT) with thin-slice (1 mm) reconstructions. The patients with documented PAVMs are at a higher risk of brain abscess, stroke, and myocardial ischemia due to a paradoxical embolism (septic, air-associated or by blood clots). Therefore, patients should be advised to receive antibiotic prophylaxis for procedures with a risk of bacteremia and to avoid scuba diving. Furthermore, clinicians should provide a long-term follow-up for patients with PAVMs to assess the growth of the untreated lesion or reperfusion of treated AVMs. The screening of liver vascular malformations (VM) is performed by Doppler ultrasound with a contrast enhancement, multiphase contrast CT scan, or contrast abdominal magnetic resonance imaging (MRI). Hepatic VMs are found in 40–70% of HHT patients [14], only patients with symptoms (including heart failure, pulmonary hypertension, abnormal cardiac biomarkers, abnormal liver function tests, abdominal pain, portal hypertension or encephalopathy require medical intervention and should be managed and followed up by a specialized center. MRI is used to screen for brain VMs. If lesions are detected, the individualized management should be carried out in a center with neurovascular expertise. For patients with anemia disproportionate to the severity of epistaxis, esophagogastroduodenoscopy (EGD) is recommended to identify suspected HHT-related bleeding. Patients who meet colorectal cancer screening criteria, and patients with SMAD4 mutations, should undergo colonoscopy. Iron deficiency and low hemoglobin counts can be caused by gastrointestinal bleeding. Therefore, the parameters should be checked regularly from the age of 35. Treatment may require the argon plasma coagulation of the gastrointestinal lesions, iron preparations, intravenous bevacizumab and/or tranexamic acid [2,10,15]. The Osler Calendar provides an overview of the necessary screening examinations, documents their results, and reminds patients of the necessary follow ups (Figure 2A). After one year of using the Osler Calendar, 76% of patients ($n = 41$) stated that they used the calendar to inform themselves about screening examinations for organ involvement in HHT (Figure 2B, left panel). The need for screening examinations was important or highly important to 48% ($n = 26$) of patients (Figure 2B, middle panel). After one year of using the Osler Calendar this number increased to 81% ($n = 44$) (Figure 2B, right panel). Furthermore, the Osler Calendar informs patients about antibiotic prophylaxis for patients with PAVMs. However, 52% ($n = 28$) of patients stated that they did not inform themselves about antibiotic prophylaxis with the Osler Calendar (Figure 2C).

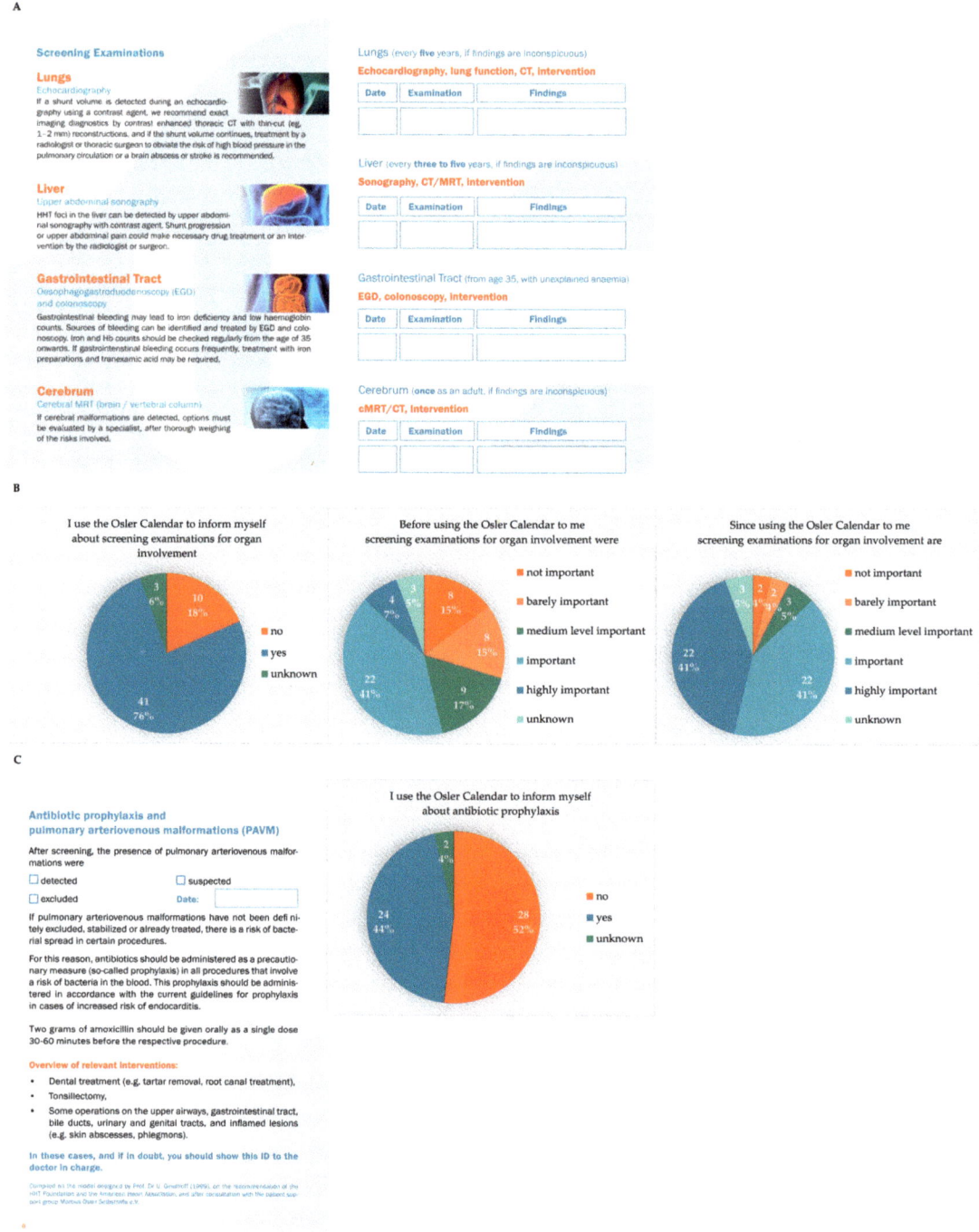

Figure 2. (**A**) Information on screening examinations for visceral lesions of HHT. (**B**) Use of the Osler Calendar for screening examinations for organ involvement. (**C**) Information on antibiotic prophylaxis.

3.3. Documentation of Epistaxis Treatment and Patient Outcome

Epistaxis is the main symptom of HHT. The intensity varies from mild, scarce bleeding to life-threatening epistaxis requiring nasal packing, hospitalization, and frequent blood transfusion, thus limiting the patient's quality of life [5]. The current therapeutic strategies follow an algorithm that takes an individualized account of the severity of epistaxis and the impairment of quality of life [1,6,16,17]. The first step is the care of the mucous membranes by the patient, as described above. The next steps in epistaxis treatment are carried out by the attending physician. Laser treatments by an otorhinolaryngologist experienced in the treatment of epistaxis in HHT are recommended [8,18–21]. The HHT foci are lasered periodically so that, ideally, only newly emergent foci remain at the initial stage. In the cases of severe epistaxis, the coagulation of the intranasal lesions can be necessary. These measures can be performed in-office by local anesthesia, but excessive bleeding can require interventions (laser therapy, coagulation and the closure of feeders, e.g., closure of the sphenopalatine artery, or sclerotherapy) under general anesthesia [16,20,22]. If those measures cannot improve the severity of epistaxis or if the involvement of other organs requires treatment, such as the gastrointestinal tract or the liver, drug therapies (tranexamic acid, bevacizumab, thalidomide and tacrolimus) are available [10,15,23–25]. The Osler Calendar documents the therapeutic measures since the last patient contact, including iron supplements, blood transfusions, nasal packing, laser therapy, coagulation, surgical interventions, and drug treatments (Figure 3A, right). As well as the therapeutic measures by the attending physician, the Osler Calendar reports the frequency of the bleeding, the average duration of the bleeding, the predominant side of the nose bleeds, the satisfaction with the current bleeding situation, the necessary interventions by the patient (nasal packing, hospitalization and previous treatments of anemia such as blood transfusions or iron supplements) and the current hemoglobin levels (Figure 3A left). The information is documented repetitively at every in-office appointment, as well as at every hospital stay. Therefore, the treatment success measured by the Epistaxis Severity Score, as well as patient satisfaction, can be traced over the course of time and treatment and can be adapted accordingly. After one year of use, 79% ($n = 43$) of patients stated that the Osler Calendar documented their therapeutic process either well or very well (Figure 3B, left panel) and 52% ($n = 28$) saw an improvement in their therapeutic process due to the documentation by the Osler Calendar (Figure 3B, right panel). Furthermore, the Osler Calendar is a tool used to inform healthcare providers about the ongoing treatment of the patient. In our study, 59% ($n = 32$) of the patients documented that their treating physicians used the Osler Calendar to inform themselves about Osler-Weber-Rendu disease (Figure 3C, left panel) and 58% ($n = 31$) of the patients reported that the Osler Calendar was used by their attending physicians for information about the therapeutic process of epistaxis treatment (Figure 3C, right panel). The overall satisfaction of the patients with the intensity and frequency of the nosebleeds in our collective of 54 patients showed a median of seven (interquartile range, IQR 5–8) on a visual analogue scale (VAS) from zero (not content at all) to ten (highly content) (Figure 3D).

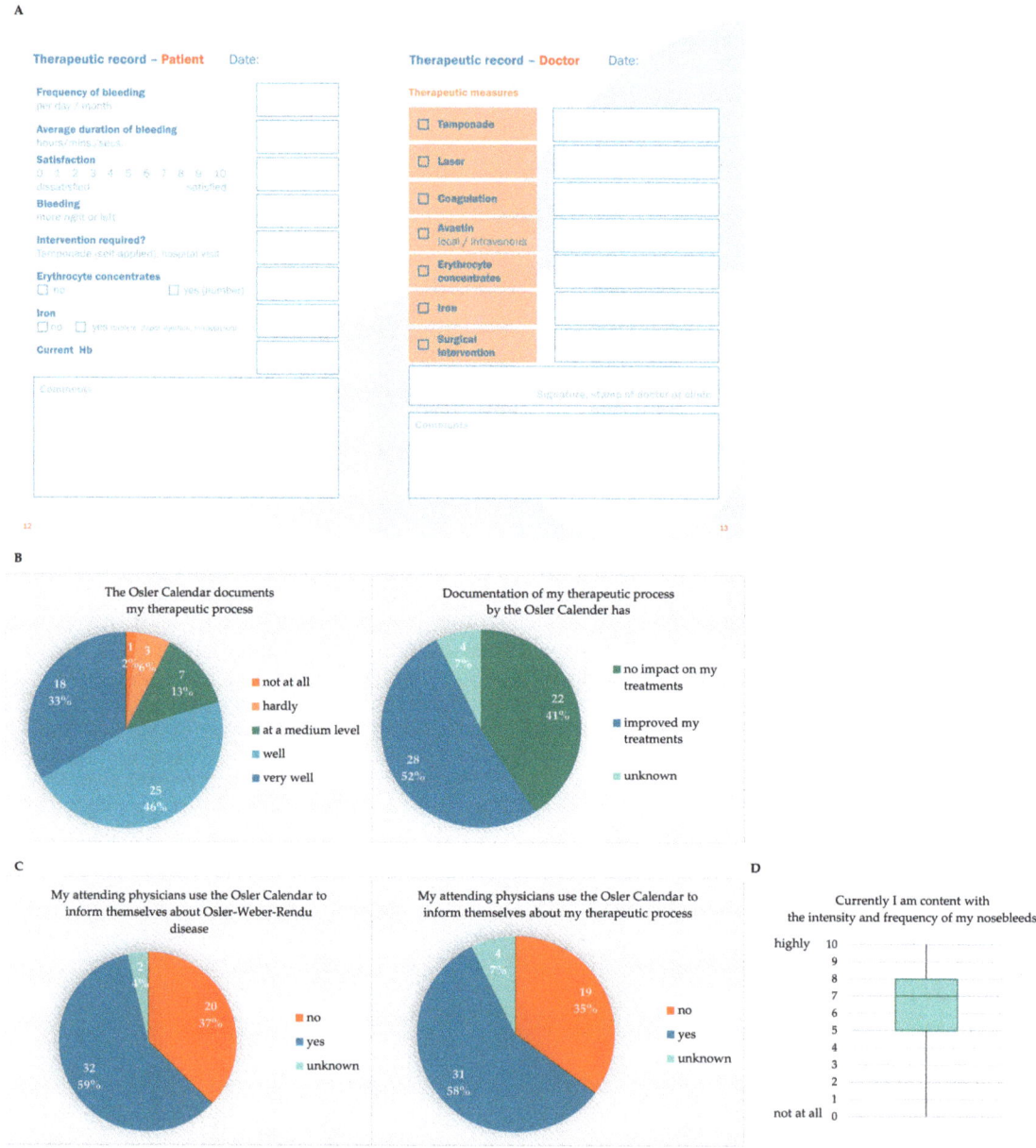

Figure 3. (**A**) Documentation of epistaxis treatment and patient outcome. (**B**) Use of the Osler Calendar for documentation of the therapeutic process. (**C**) Use of the Osler Calendar by attending physicians. (**D**) Patients' satisfaction with intensity and frequency of nosebleeds.

4. Discussion

In cancer treatment survivorship, care plans by the American Society of Clinical Oncology, consisting of treatment summaries and follow-up care plans, are well established essential components of patient care. These care plans enhance the communication between the medical team and the patient, as well as communication and coordination of care between the attending physicians and the primary care providers [26]. Following the concept of delivering patient-centered care, we developed a HHT patient care plan called the Osler Calendar to improve the communication with patients and primary care providers. Furthermore, the calendar intended to help physicians working with patients with this rare disease to recognize the importance of screening examinations and patient referral to specialized centers.

After one year of using the Osler Calendar, 85% of patients confirmed using the calendar to gain information about Osler-Weber-Rendu disease. However, only 59% of the patients documented that their primary care providers used the Osler Calendar to inform themselves about the disease and 58% about the therapeutic process of the epistaxis. The reasons for the less frequent use of the Osler Calendar by the primary care providers could be shortage of time during appointments or the missing transfer of the Osler Calendar between the patient and the primary care provider [27]. To overcome this obstacle, an electronical version of the Osler Calendar would be helpful. An app for patient education about HHT and tracking health data was previously developed [28]. In addition to information about HHT and health tracking executed by the patient, the Osler Calendar summarizes notes by the attending physician and tracks the treatment success. Therefore, the dynamic of the disease is documented and can be used to measure the effectiveness of the current therapeutic strategy. Seventy-nine percent of patients confirmed that the Osler Calendar documented their therapeutic process either well or very well and 52% even saw an improvement in their therapeutic process due to the documentation by the Osler Calendar. Similar to this result, it was reported that health tracking had a positive impact on health-related behaviors, adherence to medication or therapy, and the knowledge enhancement related to clinical procedures [29]. In the future, an app version of the calendar for iOS and Android will further improve communication with patients and primary care providers.

Next to improvement of communication, an additional objective of the Osler Calendar is to increase knowledge about HHT, treatment options, the necessary screening examinations, and the possible need for antibiotic prophylaxis. 72% of patients used the Osler Calendar for instructions about self-treatment for nosebleeds, 76% for information about screening examinations for organ involvement. The use of the Osler Calendar increased patients understanding for the need of organ screening from 48% to 81% of patients. The importance of this result is underlined by a recent study showing that the life expectancy of HHT patients systematically screened for HHT-related organ involvement is similar compared to the non-HHT control group [30]. However, only 44% of patients stated that they do inform themselves about antibiotic prophylaxis with the Osler Calendar. This number is concordant with 50% of HHT patients overall being affected by PAVMs [31]. Detailed information about the need for antibiotic prophylaxis for patients with diagnosed PAVM by the attending physician as well as patient training for nasal packing is needed to ensure correct use and patient safety [32,33].

To our knowledge, this is the first study documenting the effect of a tracking calendar for HHT used by patients and clinicians alike. The limitations of this study are the retrospective character of the analyses and the survey of patients with a non-validated questionnaire. The patient satisfaction with the ongoing treatment could be seen as biased due to the monocentric approach of the study. The study was performed at a tertiary center specialized in the treatment of HHT. The overall patient satisfaction with the intensity and frequency of the nosebleeds in the study collective of 54 patients showed a median of seven on a visual analogue scale, which was equal to the results seen in the other specialized centers using the same treatment modalities [8]. In the future, an app-based Osler Calendar used and validated by several specialized tertiary centers is needed to improve patient outcome.

5. Conclusions

In summary a patient care plan used by specialized centers, primary care providers, and the patient can provide information about the rare disease of HHT, necessary organ screening examinations, and current treatment strategies of the disease. By merging patient information and treatment plans, the optimal care for each individual patient can be achieved and patient outcome and quality of life can be improved.

Supplementary Materials: The following are available online at https://www.mdpi.com/article/10.3390/jcm10204720/s1, PDF version of the Osler Calendar, written by Caroline Seebauer, designed by Referat UK1 Regensburg University Medical Center, Regensburg, Germany. Pictures on page one and seven by adimas/Fotolia, pictures on page seven by yodiyim, Naeblys, nerthuz/Fotolia. Current version June 2019. English and German versions are available. Use, distribution, publication, replication, and demonstration of the Osler Calendar is only permitted after author's consent. For requesting permission to reproduce, reprint or translate the Osler Calendar material please contact Caroline T. Seebauer, Department of Otolaryngology, University Medical Center Regensburg, Franz-Josef-Strauß-Allee 11, 93053 Regensburg, Germany, Phone +49 941 944 9410, Email caroline.seebauer@ukr.de.

Author Contributions: C.T.S., F.E.S., C.B., T.S.K. and K.E.C.A. developed the Osler Calendar. C.T.S., R.F., T.S.K. and K.E.C.A. developed the questionnaire. C.T.S., V.F. and K.E.C.A. analyzed the data. C.T.S., V.F., F.E.S., R.F. and K.E.C.A. wrote the paper. C.B. and T.S.K. revised and edited the manuscript critically. All authors have read and agreed to the published version of the manuscript.

Funding: This research received no external funding.

Institutional Review Board Statement: The study was conducted according to the guidelines of the Declaration of Helsinki, and approved by the Ethics Committee of the University Hospital Regensburg (protocol code 17-854-101, date of approval 24-01-2018).

Informed Consent Statement: Informed consent was obtained from all subjects involved in the study.

Acknowledgments: The layout and the English translation of the Osler Calendar was designed by the Referat UK1 Externe Kommunikation (corporate communication) of the University Medical Center Regensburg. The Osler Calendar is funded by the Department of Otorhinolaryngology of the University Medical Center Regensburg. The funders had no role in study design, data collection and interpretation, or the decision to submit the work for publication.

Conflicts of Interest: The authors declare that no conflict of interest exists.

Abbreviations

AVM: arteriovenous malformations; CVM: cerebral vascular malformation; EGD: esophagogastroduodenoscopy; HHT: hereditary hemorrhagic telangiectasia; MRI: magnetic resonance imaging; PAVM: pulmonary arteriovenous malformations; CT: computed tomography; VM: vascular malformations.

References

1. Kühnel, T.; Wirsching, K.; Wohlgemuth, W.; Chavan, A.; Evert, K.; Vielsmeier, V. Hereditary Hemorrhagic Telangiectasia. *Otolaryngol. Clin. N. Am.* **2018**, *51*, 237–254. [CrossRef]
2. Faughnan, M.E.; Mager, J.J.; Hetts, S.W.; Palda, V.A.; Lang-Robertson, K.; Buscarini, E.; Deslandres, E.; Kasthuri, R.S.; Lausman, A.; Poetker, D.; et al. Second International Guidelines for the Diagnosis and Management of Hereditary Hemorrhagic Telangiectasia. *Ann. Intern. Med.* **2020**, *173*, 989–1001. [CrossRef] [PubMed]
3. Shovlin, C.L.; Buscarini, E.; Kjeldsen, A.D.; Mager, H.J.; Sabba, C.; Droege, F.; Geisthoff, U.; Ugolini, S.; Dupuis-Girod, S. European Reference Network For Rare Vascular Diseases (VASCERN) Outcome Measures For Hereditary Haemorrhagic Telangiectasia (HHT). *Orphanet J. Rare Dis.* **2018**, *13*, 136. [CrossRef]
4. Shovlin, C.L.; Guttmacher, A.E.; Buscarini, E.; Faughnan, M.E.; Hyland, R.H.; Westermann, C.J.; Kjeldsen, A.D.; Plauchu, H. Diagnostic criteria for hereditary hemorrhagic telangiectasia (Rendu-Osler-Weber syndrome). *Am. J. Med. Genet.* **2000**, *91*, 66–67. [CrossRef]
5. Wirsching, K.E.C.; Kühnel, T.S. Update on Clinical Strategies in Hereditary Hemorrhagic Telangiectasia from an ENT Point of View. *Clin. Exp. Otorhinolaryngol.* **2017**, *10*, 153–157. [CrossRef]
6. Lund, V.J.; Howard, D.J. A treatment algorithm for the management of epistaxis in hereditary hemorrhagic telangiectasia. *Am. J. Rhinol.* **1999**, *13*, 319–322. [CrossRef]

7. Wirsching, K.E.C.; Haubner, F.; Kühnel, T.S. Influence of temporary nasal occlusion (tNO) on epistaxis frequency in patients with hereditary hemorrhagic telangiectasia (HHT). *Eur. Arch. Otorhinolaryngol.* **2017**, *274*, 1891–1896. [CrossRef]
8. Bertlich, M.; Kashani, F.; Weiss, B.G.; Wiebringhaus, R.; Ihler, F.; Freytag, S.; Gires, O.; Kühnel, T.; Haubner, F. Safety and Efficacy of Blue Light Laser Treatment in Hereditary Hemorrhagic Telangiectasia. *Lasers Surg. Med.* **2021**, *53*, 309–315. [CrossRef]
9. Rohrmeier, C.; Sachs, H.G.; Kuehnel, T.S. A retrospective analysis of low dose, intranasal injected bevacizumab (Avastin) in hereditary haemorrhagic telangiectasia. *Eur. Arch. Otorhinolaryngol.* **2012**, *269*, 531–536. [CrossRef] [PubMed]
10. Chavan, A.; Schumann-Binarsch, S.; Luthe, L.; Nickau, B.; Elsässer, A.; Kühnel, T.; Geisthoff, U.; Köhne, H. Systemic therapy with bevacizumab in patients with hereditary hemorrhagic telangiectasia (HHT). *Vasa* **2013**, *42*, 106–110. [CrossRef] [PubMed]
11. Richer, S.L.; Geisthoff, U.W.; Livada, N.; Ward, P.D.; Johnson, L.; Mainka, A.; Henderson, K.J.; Maune, S.; White, R.I.; Ross, D.A. The Young's procedure for severe epistaxis from hereditary hemorrhagic telangiectasia. *Am. J. Rhinol. Allergy* **2012**, *26*, 401–404. [CrossRef]
12. López-Novoa, J.M.; Bernabeu, C. The physiological role of endoglin in the cardiovascular system. *Am. J. Physiol. Heart Circ. Physiol.* **2010**, *299*, H959–H974. [CrossRef] [PubMed]
13. Bernabeu, C.; Bayrak-Toydemir, P.; McDonald, J.; Letarte, M. Potential Second-Hits in Hereditary Hemorrhagic Telangiectasia. *J. Clin. Med.* **2020**, *9*, 3571. [CrossRef]
14. Buscarini, E.; Gandolfi, S.; Alicante, S.; Londoni, C.; Manfredi, G. Liver involvement in hereditary hemorrhagic telangiectasia. *Abdom. Radiol.* **2018**, *43*, 1920–1930. [CrossRef] [PubMed]
15. Geisthoff, U.W.; Seyfert, U.T.; Kübler, M.; Bieg, B.; Plinkert, P.K.; König, J. Treatment of epistaxis in hereditary hemorrhagic telangiectasia with tranexamic acid—A double-blind placebo-controlled cross-over phase IIIB study. *Thromb. Res.* **2014**, *134*, 565–571. [CrossRef]
16. Kuan, E.C.; Peng, K.A.; Thompson, C.F.; Suh, J.D.; Wang, M.B. Sinonasal quality of life outcomes following laser treatment of epistaxis related to hereditary hemorrhagic telangiectasia. *Lasers Med. Sci.* **2017**, *32*, 527–531. [CrossRef] [PubMed]
17. Poje, G.; Kavanagh, M.M. Hereditary hemorrhagic telangiectasia-laser treatment of epistaxis. *Ear. Nose Throat J.* **2017**, *96*, E10–E14.
18. Wu, V.; Kell, E.; Faughnan, M.E.; Lee, J.M. In-Office KTP Laser for Treating Hereditary Hemorrhagic Telangiectasia–Associated Epistaxis. *Laryngoscope* **2021**, *131*, E689–E693. [CrossRef]
19. Sautter, N.B.; Smith, T.L. Treatment of Hereditary Hemorrhagic Telangiectasia–Related Epistaxis. *Otolaryngol. Clin. N. Am.* **2016**, *49*, 639–654. [CrossRef]
20. Geisthoff, U.; Fiorella, M.; Fiorella, R. Treatment of Recurrent Epistaxis in HHT. *Curr. Pharm. Des.* **2006**, *12*, 1237–1242. [CrossRef]
21. Jørgensen, G.; Lange, B.; Wanscher, J.H.; Kjeldsen, A.D. Efficiency of laser treatment in patients with hereditary hemorrhagic telangiectasia. *Eur. Arch. Otorhinolaryngol.* **2011**, *268*, 1765–1770. [CrossRef]
22. Marcos, S.; Botella, L.M.; Albiñana, V.; Arbia, A.; de Rosales, A.M. Sclerotherapy on Demand with Polidocanol to Treat HHT Nosebleeds. *J. Clin. Med.* **2021**, *10*, 3845. [CrossRef] [PubMed]
23. Chavan, A.; Schumann-Binarsch, S.; Schmuck, B.; Oltmer, F.; Geisthoff, U.; Hoppe, F.; Wirsching, K.; Klempnauer, J.; Manns, M.; Philip Thomas, R.; et al. Emerging role of bevacizumab in management of patients with symptomatic hepatic involvement in Hereditary Hemorrhagic Telangiectasia. *Am. J. Hematol.* **2017**, *92*, E641–E644. [CrossRef]
24. Sommer, N.; Droege, F.; Gamen, K.E.; Geisthoff, U.; Gall, H.; Tello, K.; Richter, M.J.; Deubner, L.M.; Schmiedel, R.; Hecker, M.; et al. Treatment with low-dose tacrolimus inhibits bleeding complications in a patient with hereditary hemorrhagic telangiectasia and pulmonary arterial hypertension. *Pulm. Circ.* **2018**, *9*, 2045894018805406. [CrossRef]
25. Buscarini, E.; Botella, L.M.; Geisthoff, U.; Kjeldsen, A.D.; Mager, H.J.; Pagella, F.; Suppressa, P.; Zarrabeitia, R.; Dupuis-Girod, S.; Shovlin, C.L. Safety of thalidomide and bevacizumab in patients with hereditary hemorrhagic telangiectasia. *Orphanet J. Rare Dis.* **2019**, *14*, 28. [CrossRef]
26. Mayer, D.K.; Nekhlyudov, L.; Snyder, C.F.; Merrill, J.K.; Wollins, D.S.; Shulman, L.N. American Society of Clinical Oncology clinical expert statement on cancer survivorship care planning. *J. Oncol. Pract.* **2014**, *10*, 345–351. [CrossRef]
27. Von dem Knesebeck, O.; Koens, S.; Marx, G.; Scherer, M. Perceptions of time constraints among primary care physicians in Germany. *BMC Fam. Pract.* **2019**, *20*, 142. [CrossRef] [PubMed]
28. My HHT Tracker App-CureHHT. Available online: https://curehht.org/understanding-hht/get-support/my-hht-tracker-app/ (accessed on 16 August 2021).
29. Han, M.; Lee, E. Effectiveness of Mobile Health Application Use to Improve Health Behavior Changes: A Systematic Review of Randomized Controlled Trials. *Healthc. Inform. Res.* **2018**, *24*, 207–226. [CrossRef] [PubMed]
30. de Gussem, E.M.; Kroon, S.; Hosman, A.E.; Kelder, J.C.; Post, M.C.; Snijder, R.J.; Mager, J.J. Hereditary Hemorrhagic Telangiectasia (HHT) and Survival: The Importance of Systematic Screening and Treatment in HHT Centers of Excellence. *J. Clin. Med.* **2020**, *9*, 3581. [CrossRef] [PubMed]
31. Majumdar, S.; McWilliams, J.P. Approach to Pulmonary Arteriovenous Malformations: A Comprehensive Update. *J. Clin. Med.* **2020**, *9*, 1927. [CrossRef]
32. Velthuis, S.; Buscarini, E.; Gossage, J.R.; Snijder, R.J.; Mager, J.J.; Post, M.C. Clinical implications of pulmonary shunting on saline contrast echocardiography. *J. Am. Soc. Echocardiogr.* **2015**, *28*, 255–263. [CrossRef] [PubMed]
33. Droege, F.; Lueb, C.; Thangavelu, K.; Stuck, B.A.; Lang, S.; Geisthoff, U. Nasal self-packing for epistaxis in Hereditary Hemorrhagic Telangiectasia increases quality of life. *Rhinology* **2019**, *57*, 231–239. [CrossRef] [PubMed]

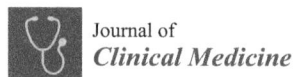

Article

Sclerotherapy on Demand with Polidocanol to Treat HHT Nosebleeds

Sol Marcos [1,*], Luisa María Botella [2], Virginia Albiñana [2], Agustina Arbia [1] and Anna María de Rosales [3]

[1] Otorhinolaringology Department, Hospital Universitario Fundación Alcorcón, 28922 Madrid, Spain; roagusdi@gmail.com
[2] CIBER Rare Diseases Unit 707, Centro de Investigaciones Biológicas Margarita Salas, CSIC, 28040 Madrid, Spain; cibluisa@cib.csic.es (L.M.B.); vir_albi_di@yahoo.es (V.A.)
[3] Pharmaceutical Department, Hospital Universitario Fundación Alcorcón, 28922 Madrid, Spain; annamariamrc@gmail.com
* Correspondence: solmarsal70@gmail.com

Abstract: Epistaxis is the most prevalent clinical symptom in Hereditary Haemorrhagic Telangiectasia (HHT), causing anaemia and decreasing the quality of life (QOL). Since 2013, in Hospital Universitario Fundación Alcorcón, more than 150 HHT patients have been treated by nose sclerotherapy on demand. This study shows the results of 105 patients treated with sclerotherapy between 2017 and 2019. HHT-ESS (epistaxis severity score) was used to measure the severity and frequency of epistaxis. QOL was determined before and after treatment by EuroQol-5D (EQ-5D) and the visual analogue scale (VAS) on the health condition. According to HHT-ESS before treatment, 22 patients presented mild, 35 moderate, and 47 severe epistaxes. Sclerotherapy significantly decreased the frequency and severity of epistaxis, with a significant drop of HHT-ESS in 4.6 points, from 6.23 ± 2.3 to 1.64 ± 1.6. Furthermore, the QOL significantly improved, the EQ-5D scale raised from 0.7 ± 0.26 pre- to 0.92 ± 0.16 post-treatment ($p < 0.05$). Additionally, VAS mean value showed a significant increase from 4.38 ± 2.4 to 8.35 ± 1.2. The QOL improvement was correlated with the ESS decrease. In conclusion, this study shows that on-demand sclerotherapy at the office significantly reduces HHT epistaxis as well as improved the patients' QOL.

Keywords: HHT; epistaxis; sclerotherapy; polidocanol; propranolol; HHT-ESS; quality of life

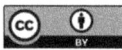

1. Introduction

Hereditary haemorrhagic telangiectasia (HHT), also known as Rendu–Osler–Weber disease, is an autosomal dominant multisystemic vascular disorder with incomplete penetrance. The estimated prevalence ranges from 1:5000 to 1:8000 [1], and it is thus considered a rare disease.

HHT affects several organs and is therefore the cause of a wide variety of clinical manifestations. The diagnosis for HHT is achieved by the Curaçao criteria [2]: epistaxis, mucocutaneous telangiectases, first-degree family inheritance, and visceral arteriovenous malformations (AVM). The presence of three of these four criteria results in a conclusive HHT diagnosis. Positive genetic tests are definitive for the diagnosis, being especially useful for young patients that have not yet developed clinical manifestations, according to Curaçao criteria [3]. Affected individuals display a variety of vascular malformations from telangiectases (dilated and very fragile capillaries) to AVMs. Telangiectases are usually present in the nasal mucosa but also on the lips, tongue, and on the tip of the fingers. There are vascular lesions in the gastrointestinal (GI) tract, AVMs on the liver, lungs, and more rarely (less than 10%) on the Central Nervous System. Typical lesions exhibit markedly dilated, tortuous venules with absent or abnormal muscle walls, frequently directly linked to unusually dilated arterioles [4]. On the nasal epithelium, telangiectases with thin walls are exposed to breathing air trauma, leading to dryness and nasal crusting. Damage causes rupture of these vessels and the lack of functional elastic fibres prevents normal vasoconstriction; thus, haemorrhage becomes difficult to handle. In an online survey of 666 HHT patients, 97% stated daily nosebleeds, and 49% received invasive treatments to control the haemorrhages [4]. Continuous bleeding can result in anaemia with the need for iron therapy and eventually blood transfusions.

In another questionnaire, among 220 HHT patients, about 50% suffered from daily bleeding, and 76.5% had nosebleeds at least once a week [5]. Nose bleeding in HHT requires quick actions, from nasal packing with absorbable materials to more invasive procedures and even hospitalisations [5]. Nosebleeds severity often becomes worse with age, impairing a patient's normal life. Chronic anaemia leads to continuous visits to the hospital, blood transfusions, invasive procedures, and hospitalisations. All these situations have a significant detrimental impact on the HHT patients' quality of life (QOL) [6].

Epistaxis is the most frequent clinical manifestation (more than 90% of HHT patients). Prevention for mild recurrent bleeding requires careful cleaning and moisturising of nasal nostrils. A variety of topical and oral drugs have been used for therapy: hormones such as estriol; selective estrogen receptor modulators such as tamoxifen or raloxifene; antifibrinolytics such as tranexamic acid (showing anti-inflammatory proprieties); and antiangiogenic agents such as propranolol or bevacizumab [7]. HHT management needs multidisciplinary assistance. Recurrent or severe epistaxis should be referred to an otorhinolaryngologist for local control and followed by blood tests to evaluate the need for oral or IV iron supplementation or blood transfusions to treat anaemia.

Management of epistaxis in HHT patients is different from non-HHT. A nosebleed can be the most predominant and incapacitating symptom in the elderly. Unfortunately, there is no agreement on which is the best type of treatment. Nasal packing can lead to more severe bleeding when removed, and cauterisation not only can worsen the lesions but also carries a risk of septal perforation. There are numerous treatments, including laser, radiofrequency, sclerotherapy, embolisation, and surgical procedures. Nevertheless, none is perfect, and most of them show limited efficacy, especially in severe cases.

Different treatments are applied depending on the frequency and severity of epistaxis. A nosebleed is often an emergency, but its management is also determined by the clinician's experience. For recurrent nose bleedings, ENT specialists can perform several forms of laser photocoagulation (CO_2, argon, neodymium-doped yttrium aluminium garnet (Nd-YAG), flashlamp-pulsed dye, and potassium titanyl phosphate (KTP)), plasma coagulation or surgical micro-debridement. More invasive surgery options involve septodermoplasty and full nasal closure (Young's procedure) [3]. Arterial embolisation is performed for severe emergency bleeding. Surgical procedures have shown the highest efficiency as they treat the bleeding in its origin; however, they are not exempt from complications such as crusting, bad smell, scarring, and obligatory mouth breathing. The success of these techniques is not complete nor permanent, and surgery is not appropriated in cases of mild or moderate epistaxis [1].

Local sclerotherapy consists of submucosal or subperichondrial injections of polidocanol, an agent causing obstruction of the blood flow and clotting and collapse of the lesion. Sclerotherapy is an established treatment for AVM (varicose veins) and bleedings of the GI and of the genitourinary tract. It has been used in angiomas in the head and neck but is not standardised for HHT. A review of this technique was published by Dr. Morais using submucosal injections of polidocanol. He performed nearly 300 injections in 45 patients for 15 years [8]. Nosebleeds improved both in frequency and quantity in 95% of the cases, and no relevant side effects were reported. More recently, sclerotherapy has been used with satisfactory results by Boyer et al. [6]. Thus, sclerotherapy should be considered as an alternative to surgical procedures, with the advantage of its reduced aggressiveness and low risks derived from it.

2. Materials and Methods

2.1. Patients and Study Design

This work represents a cross-sectional study performed between 2017 and 2019. It includes HHT patients treated with sclerotherapy at the Hospital Universitario Fundación Alcorcón (HUFA). Before this study, in 2017, we conducted another cross-sectional study on 38 HHT patients treated with sclerotherapy and topical propranolol [9]. That first study was continued and updated in 2019, scaling up to a total of 105 patients. All patients were older than 18 years, had a confirmed diagnosis of HHT (clinical and/or genetic), and were followed by the HUFA Otorhinolaryngology Unit.

Patients underwent a general clinical screening: variables such as gender, frequency of epistaxis, previous and current medical treatment for epistaxis, and the length of time they were under sclerotherapy treatment were recorded. Specific otorhinolaryngologist examination (anterior rhinoscopy and endoscopy) was always performed by the same otorhinolaryngologist specialist in HHT. Telangiectases were described by their morphological characteristics [10] according to Zarrabeitia's classification: absence of telangiectases (0); isolate punctuated telangiectases (I); multiple punctuated telangiectases (II); ramified telangiectases (III); isolate complex vascular malformations (IVa); multiple complex vascular malformations (IVb).

As inclusion criteria, patients should not have received polidocanol sclerotherapy at least in the 4 weeks prior to the study. The study received approval from the Pharmaceutical Committee and the Clinical Research Ethics Committee from HUFA.

Exclusion criteria included patients under 18 years of age, Young's complete nasal closure, and allergies to polidocanol or its excipients.

2.2. Outcomes and Assessments

The primary outcome was the impact on frequency and severity of epistaxis, as measured by the HHT epistaxis severity score (HHT-ESS). HHT-ESS is an objective, standardised and internationally validated reference tool to estimate the severity of epistaxis in HHT patients [11]. HHT-ESS is calculated from six parameters related to epistaxis: frequency, duration, and intensity of nosebleed, presence/absence of anaemia, need for blood transfusion, and need to seek medical care to treat the haemorrhage.

In this study, the baseline as reference was 4 weeks before starting the treatment and at least 4 weeks after the last session of sclerotherapy. The ESS scale ranges from 0 (absence of epistaxis) to 10. The scores indicates that from 0 to 1 is considered inside the normality range, from 1 to 4 nosebleed is classified as mild, from 4 to 7 is moderate, and from 7 to 10 the haemorrhage is severe, not only searching medical assistance but also being associated with anaemia and requiring blood transfusions. No serious adverse events to the treatment were reported. Any new symptom not present at the baseline was tracked.

Patient's QOL before and after treatment was assessed by EuroQol-5D-3L (EQ-5D) scale [12]. This scale ranges from 0 (the worst situation—death) to 1 (the best health status). In addition, a visual analogue scale (VAS) which estimates (QOL) with a value from 0 (the worst health status) to 10 (the best health status), was included. For this study, approval from local Clinical Research Ethics Committee was received, and for the inclusion of each patient, informed consent was required.

2.3. Sclerotherapy with Polidocanol 1%

Patients were attended at the office, on-demand. The criteria to treat them were recurrent and/or gushing or pouring nosebleeds. Patients contacted the ENT specialist when their nosebleed required care, either for its frequency or its severity. Patients were immediately attended as soon as possible, or with a maximum waiting time of 2 days.

The procedure started with the administration of topical anaesthesia (lidocaine 1% and adrenaline) to numb the area. To minimise the discomfort of the treatment, the anaesthetic is left in place for at least 10 min, usually more. The adrenaline helps not only to decrease the bleeding but it also helps with the identification of the telangiectases: the mucosa becomes paler while the telangiectases stay red due to the impairment of the elastic fibres and the muscular layer on their walls. Once identified, the polidocanol (1%) is injected in small volumes with a 1 mL syringe and a 30 G needle (25 G when the lesions are farther into the nasal cavity and a longer needle is required). The quantity of liquid varies according to the tolerance of the patient and the size of the lesions; usually, the first injections are the most painful, as topical anaesthesia just numbs the area. The procedure (infiltration) is repeated as many times as needed, though never on both sides of the septum at the same time to avoid septum perforations. The administration takes place with different 1 mL syringes and 30 G needles. After the procedure, residual bleeding is controlled with a self-absorbent packing (e.g., Surgicel or similar). Finally, patients receive prophylactic antibiotic treatment, either topically (terramycin ointment, tobramycin or gentamycin drops) or systemically (doxycycline), administered every 12 h for 1 week. Following sclerotherapy, propranolol is used as a topical nasal ointment (0.5% propranolol in Vaseline) prepared at the Hospital Pharmacy as a maintenance treatment to space the time between sclerotherapies.

2.4. Statistical Analysis

For data analysis, the SPSS17 program was used. The data are described by absolute and relative frequencies for qualitative variables and by the mean and standard deviation (SD) for quantitative variables according to data distribution. To analyse the change in the dichotomous variables, McNemar asymmetry test was used, and to analyse the change of quantitative variables, the t-Student test of repeated measures, the Chi-square test, and the non-parametric Wilcoxon test were used. All tests are considered bilateral and as significant when the p-value < 0.05 or lower.

3. Results

A total of 150 HHT patients were treated and evaluated between March 2017 and May 2019, but only 105 completed the study. Missing data were due to a lack of filling the patient's diary, lack of adherence to treatment, or non-acceptance to enter the study. A total of 59% (n = 62) were women, and the average age was 54.6 ± 14.0 years. All HHT patients in the study presented nasal telangiectases and epistaxis (100.0%). At baseline, patients showed either isolated or multiple telangiectases in nostrils. Complex malformations were common in most of our patients. More than 50% of the patients presented grade IVb lesions according to Zarrabeitia's classification on the nasal mucosa [10].

Due to the extension and the complex macroscopic characteristics of the telangiectases, many patients needed several sclerotherapy sessions to control the symptoms. The duration of each session would depend on the clinic, the complexity and extension of the lesions, the bleeding during the procedure, the endurance to pain and the patient physical and psychological status. The nose is a sensitive organ, and some of the injections, especially those in the lateral wall, the turbinates, or the valve, in spite of topical anaesthesia, are quite painful. The frequency of the visits is also dependent on the bilateral affectation since it is not advised to treat both sides of the septum at the same time.

3.1. HHT Epistaxis Severity Score

Baseline mean HHT-ESS pre-treatment was 6.23 ± 2.32 and decreased significantly after-treatment to 1.64 ± 1.6 (p < 0.05) (Figure 1A). In the 22 patients with mild ESS, the improvement was 2.1 points (from 2.79 before treatment to 0.7 after sclerotherapy); in the 35 patients with moderate EES, the improvement was 4.12 points (from 5.52 pre to 1.4 post), and in the 47 patients with severe epistaxis, the mean improvement of their ESS achieved 6.1 points (from 8.4 pre- to 2.3 post-treatment). These differences were statistically significant (p < 0.001) in all the groups. When all the severity groups were considered together, differences between before and after treatment were also highly significant (Figure 1B).

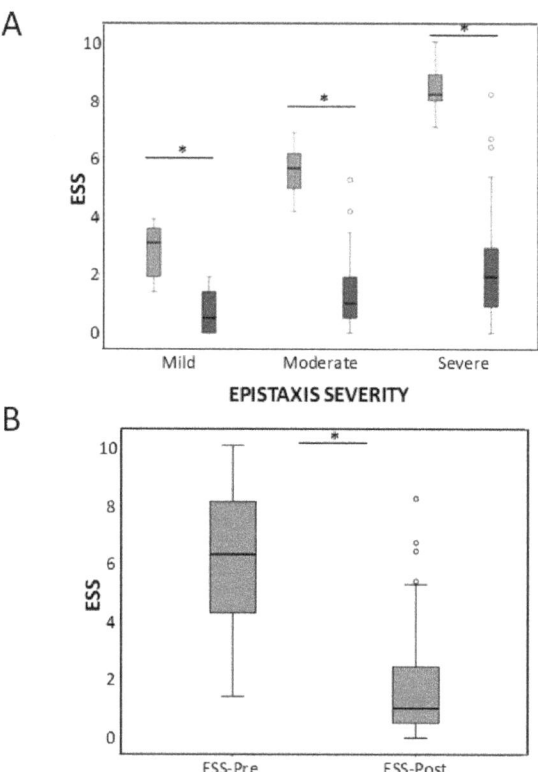

Figure 1. (**A**) Box-whiskers plots corresponding to the HHT-ESS in mild, moderate, and severe HHT patients before and after the sclerotherapy treatment. * $p < 0.001$. (**B**) Considering all the severity groups together, differences between before and after treatment were also highly significant * $p < 0.001$.

Then, each of the parameters conforming to the HHT-ESS was individually analysed. All the six factors of the HHT-ESS pre- and post-treatment were significantly reduced.

Regarding epistaxis frequency (Figure 2A), at baseline, 41.9% (44) of patients had several epistaxes daily, 10.5% at least once a day, 31.4% several times per week, 12.4% once a week, and only 4 patients (3.8%) referred to bleedings as once a month. There was no patient referring less than once a month bleeding. However, after the sclerotherapy, only 6 patients (5.7%) still had nosebleeds several times per day, 12 patients (11.4%) several times per week, 25.7% once a week, 24.8% once a month, and 34 patients (32.4%) less than once a month (Figure 2A). The length of the nosebleeds is shown in Figure 2B. Before treatment, bleeding was longer than 30 min in 19% of our patients, 23.8% were bleeding between 16 and 30 min, 28% from 6 to 15 min, (27.6%) from 1 to 5 min, and just 1 patient was bleeding less than a minute. After sclerotherapy, just 1 patient had nosebleeds longer than 15 min, 11 patients (10.5%) from 6 to 15 min, 41 patients (39%) from 1 to 5 min, and 52 patients (49.5%) had less than 1-min nosebleeds (Figure 2B).

The intensity of the nosebleed was described as gushing or pouring by 72 patients (68.6%) and non-gushing by 31.4% before treatment (Figure 3). After treatment, only 6 patients (5.7%) still had gushing nosebleeds, while the majority, 99 patients (94.3%), described their haemorrhages as non-gushing. This difference was statistically significant ($p < 0.001$) (Figure 3). In 67 patients (63.8%), medical attention was needed because of nosebleeds before the sclerotherapy treatment (Figure 4). After the sclerotherapy, only 13 patients (12.4%) needed medical attention (Figure 4). This difference was statistically significant comparing before and after treatment ($p < 0.001$).

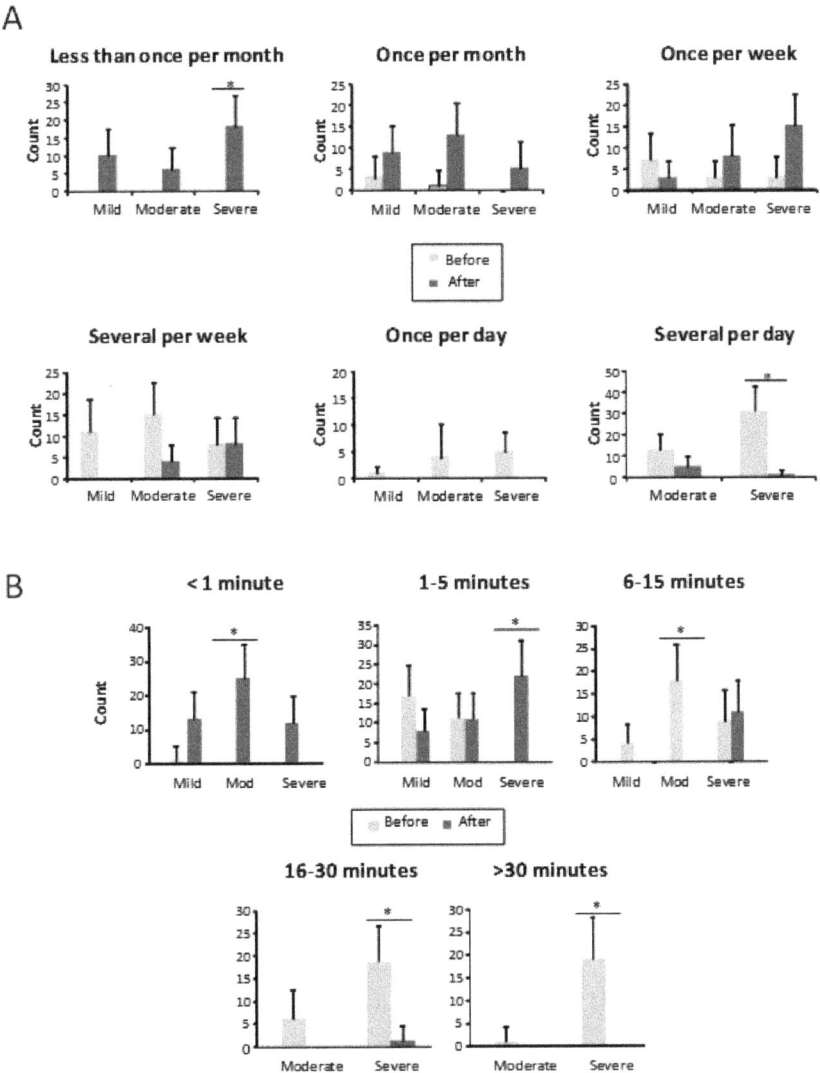

Figure 2. (**A**) Frequency of epistaxis, in the different groups, before and after the treatment in mild, moderate, and severe HHT-ESS patients. * $p < 0.05$. (**B**) Bleeding time of patients in each class, before and after the treatment in mild, moderate, and severe HHT-ESS patients. * $p < 0.05$.

Finally, the results concerning anaemia and blood transfusions are shown in Figure 5A. A total of 74 patients (70.5%) were anaemic before treatment (2 in the mild ESS group, 29 in the moderate one, and 43 in the severe group). After the treatment, only 19 patients (18.1%) (4 from the moderate HHT-ESS group and 15 from the severe one) were still anaemic. This difference was statistically significant ($p < 0.001$) (Figure 5A). A number of 31 patients (29.5%), all of them in the severe HHT-ESS group, had received blood transfusions because of anaemia by nosebleeds. After the sclerotherapy, only eight patients (7.6%) still needed blood transfusions (Figure 5B).

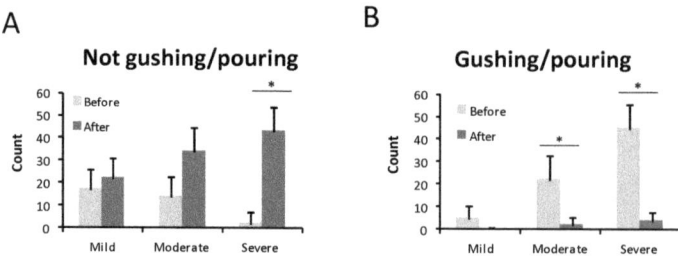

Figure 3. Type of bleeding before and after the treatment in mild, moderate, and severe HHT-ESS patients. (**A**). Not gushing/pouring. (**B**). Gushing/pouring. * $p < 0.05$.

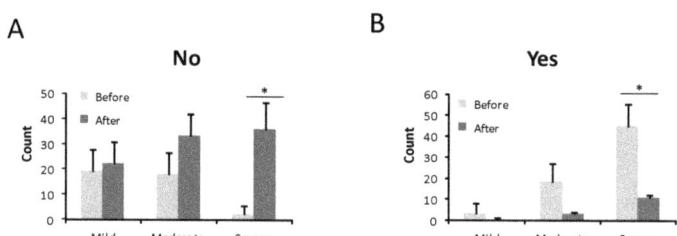

Figure 4. Number of patients who needed medical care before and after the treatment in mild, moderate, and severe HHT-ESS patients. (**A**). No need medical care. (**B**). Need medical care. * $p < 0.05$.

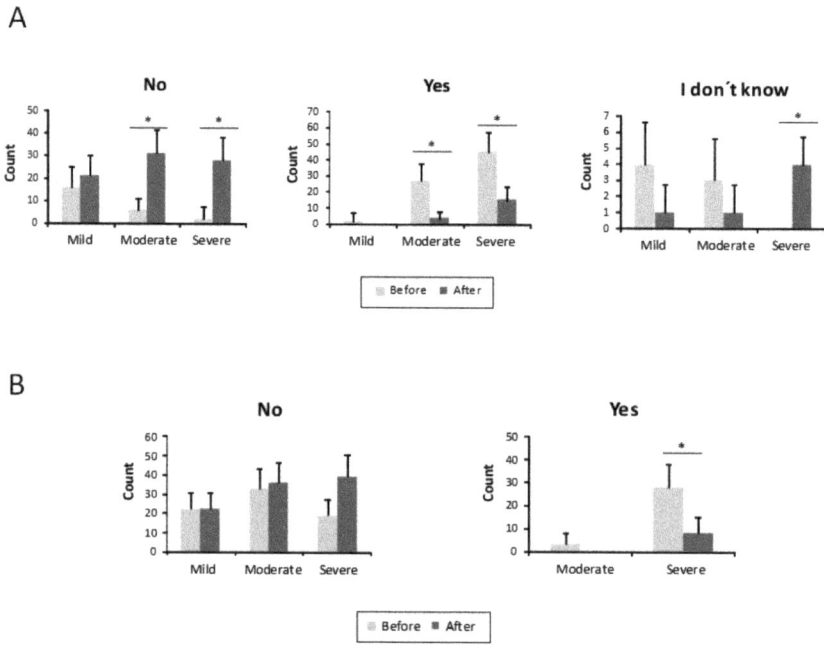

Figure 5. Parameters related to anaemia from the HHT-ESS. (**A**) Number of patients is represented with, without anaemia, or without anaemia test, before and after the treatment in mild, moderate, and severe HHT patients. (**B**) The need for transfusions in the same groups of patients is shown before and after the treatment. * $p < 0.05$.

3.2. Results of the QOL Measurements

QOL was measured by two scales—EQ-5D and VAS. In both cases, the results improved, as shown in Figure 6A,B, respectively. The results measured by the EQ-5D scale improved significantly from 0.7 ± 0.26 before treatment to 0.92 ± 0.16 after treatment $p < 0.05$. Every dimension of the scale increased its value, observing the highest difference in daily activity and psychological parameters such as and anxiety/depression (Figure 6A). When completing the EQ-5D pre-treatment, the patient had to evaluate his/her health status prior to the beginning of the sclerotherapy. For the EQ-5D post-treatment, the patients' answers had to reflect their current status. The statistical analysis applied was a paired t-Student test between pre- and post-treatment data. The mean difference on the EQ-5D before and after treatment was 0.22 ± 0.25. This difference was statistically significant ($p < 0.05$) with a confidence interval of 95% (IC 0.27 ± 0.17). Taking into account each parameter in the EQ-5D, the following results are observed:

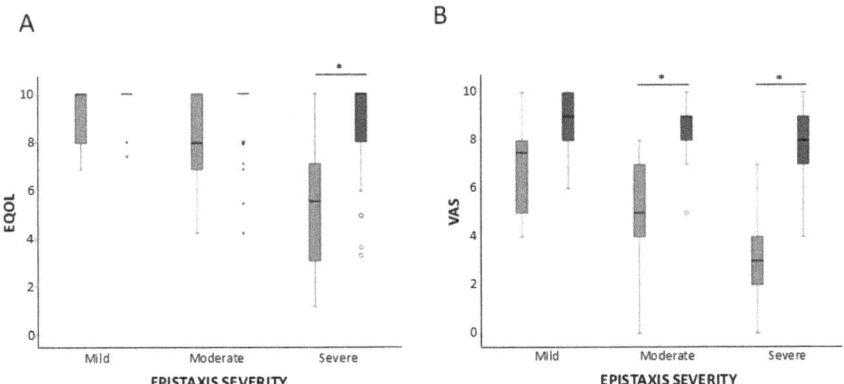

Figure 6. Box-whiskers plots corresponding to QOL parameters, EQ-5D (**A**) and VAS (**B**). Results are shown before and after the treatment in mild, moderate, and severe HHT-ESS patients. * $p < 0.05$.

EQ-5D Mobility: at baseline, 25% of patients complained of mobility problems. After the treatment, only 8% still had mobility problems. This difference was statistically significant (chi-square test $p < 0.0001$).

EQ-5D personal care: at baseline, 16% of patients had some trouble dressing or washing. After treatment, only 3% referred problems. This difference was statistically significant (chi-square test $p < 0.0001$).

EQ-5D daily activities: before treatment, 9% of patients declared they were unable to perform normal daily activities, and 51% had some kind of impairment. After the sclerotherapy, only 1% was still unable to complete their chores, and 13% had some impairment, while 86% of the patient referred no trouble at all. This difference was statistically significant (chi-square test $p < 0.0001$).

EQ-5D pain/discomfort: at baseline, 4% of patients complained of severe pain or discomfort and 40% of patients referred moderate pain or discomfort. After treatment, just 1% still had severe pain/discomfort and 12% moderate pain/discomfort; 87% of patients had no pain or discomfort. These answers showed an improvement of 67%, which was statistically significant (chi-square test $p < 0.001$).

EQ-5D anxiety/depression: at baseline, 21% of patients were very anxious or depressed, and 34% referred to moderate anxiety or depression. After treatment, 2% still had severe anxiety/depression and 17% still were moderately anxious/depressed; 81% of patients were fine. A total of 41% of the severe cases improved to moderate, and 50% of the moderate anxious/depressed patients had a complete recovery. This difference was statistically significant (chi-square test $p < 0.001$).

VAS is a descriptive self-evaluation scale of health status. VAS is also designed to measure QOL, 0 being the worst and 10 being the best score. An increase in the VAS scale from 4.48 ± 2.4 before to 8.35 ± 1.25) after the treatment was observed, and it was statistically significant ($p < 0.05$) (Figure 6B). The mean difference on the VAS scale before and after treatment was 3.87 ± 2.36, 1.81 ± 1.5 in the mild group, 3.5 ± 2.02 in the moderate group, and 4.12 ± 1.48. This difference was statistically significant ($p < 0.001$) for all the groups.

4. Discussion

The results presented in this study s demonstrate that on-demand sclerotherapy with polidocanol is a highly effective therapy, not only in reducing the severity of bleedings in the HHT population according to the HHT-ESS score but also in improving their QOL. All patients showed a drop in the HHT-ESS value before and after the sclerotherapy.

The minimal important difference (MID) of ESS in HHT patients was calculated by Yin et al. [13] as 0.71 to be clinically significant. In our study, the mean decrease achieved was 4.58 ± 2.3 points (2.1 in our 22 mild epistaxis group, 4.1 in the 36 patients with moderate nosebleeds, and 6.1 in the 47 subjects with severe bleedings). Interestingly, this decrease represents the highest ESS score drop recorded until now in the literature in a large group of patients.

Prior to treatment, most of our patients were classified as suffering from severe epistaxis according to their HHT-ESS. More than 90% of them ($n = 101$) had more than one bleeding episode per week. Among them, 41.9%, referred several episodes per day. These data are similar to the baseline score in the Whitehead et al. [14] cohort, who participated from 2011 to 2015 in the NOSE clinical trial study, to evaluate the safety and efficacy of different nasal sprays (bevacizumab 1%, estriol 0.1%, tranexamic 10%, and saline serum as placebo). In Whitehead et al., no significant differences were observed before and after treatments compared to placebo, according to the HHT-ESS. However, in our work, all the variables composing the HHT-ESS scale were significantly decreased. After the sclerotherapy procedure, only six patients continued bleeding several times a day.

The EQ-5D is a valid method to assess the impact of nosebleeds on the QOL of HHT patients. Our results show that those items with a larger number of affected patients before treatment (mainly daily activities and anxiety/depression) were the ones improving more after treatment. The same holds true for the VAS scale. A linear correlation between the HHT-ESS decrease and the increase in the QOL scales is detected.

The recovery of the QOL in our patients, evaluated by both EQ-5D and VAS, is remarkable. The anxiety/depression item is the dimension showing a better improvement in our patients after the treatment. The majority (58%) of patients referred psychological problems at baseline, and only 18 (19%) complained about their emotional state after the treatment. This improvement is in line with the reduction of the HHT-ESS. Bleeding and weakness due to anaemia affect the anxiety/depression state. The decrease in bleeding and the improvement in the anaemic condition helps to strengthen the psychological state of the patients.

The baseline QOL score in the Zarrabeitia et al. [15] cohort was better than in our population. The dimensions of daily activities and anxiety/depression of EQ-5D were impaired in 60% and 54.3%, respectively, in our patients was 24.6%, and 43.9% in the Zarrabeitia et al. [15] group. Moreover, baseline VAS values scored 7.37 points, while our baseline VAS mean value was 4.48 points. Thus, even when the QOL of our cohort was more severely affected, the improvement following sclerotherapy was remarkable.

Boyer et al. [6] performed sclerotherapy with sodium tetradecyl sulphate in a cross-sectional study evaluated for a period of 12 weeks. A significant reduction of 0.95 points on the HHT-ESS scale ($p = 0.027$) was observed. The fact that our results are far better may be attributed to the time of follow-up. Patients may require several sessions of sclerotherapy to achieve good control of their haemorrhages, and 12 weeks might not be enough. A longer follow-up allows the ENT to monitor the appearance of new lesions and to perform new sclerotherapy procedures on-demand upon nosebleeds recurrences.

Side effects of sclerotherapy in our group are either negligible or non-existing. If we compare our study to surgical procedures, the risk/benefit complications are highly favourable in our case. With drugs, such as thalidomide, the safety profile is rather unfavourable for thalidomide. Thalidomide cannot be administered without interruption due to its adverse events, peripheral neuropathy, among others [16]. On the other hand, upon treatment discontinuation, a considerable rebound effect appears.

In the case of bevacizumab, the cost-effectiveness is favourable to polidocanol, though the injection of bevacizumab and cyanoacrylate glue sounds promising [17], showing improvement in 31 patients with moderate-severe epistaxis after a mean follow up of 26.6 months (interval from 9 to 56). From a baseline HHT-ESS of 7.8 before injection, it decreased to 3.8 after the treatments. It is a line of treatment worth watching.

After more than 8 years of sclerotherapy practice in HHT patients, we must say that in our hands, the treatment is safe, with good tolerance and with hardly any relevant adverse effects.

Limitations of the Study

This study has important limitations. Clinical manifestations are distinct in different HHT patients, and they usually worsen with age. Epistaxis is the most common symptom, but there are many more (pulmonary involvement, digestive issues, hepatic lesions, strokes, and internal bleeding). We have only evaluated the changes related to the ENT field. Patients demanded the otorhinolaryngology consultation, and their treatment was scheduled on-demand based on their epistaxis symptoms. The distance to the hospital represents one limitation, especially in severe cases or older patients, when travelling becomes a challenge.

5. Conclusions

Sclerotherapy does not represent a definite cure for nosebleeds. However, it supposes an improvement not only on epistaxis but also on clinically related issues such as anaemia and psychological status) and, consequently, on the QOL.

Many patients manifest their satisfaction overtly on the treatment and the positive influence on their lives. This study demonstrates that on-demand sclerotherapy performed at the office significantly reduces HHT epistaxis and greatly improves the patients' QOL.

Author Contributions: S.M., L.M.B., V.A., A.A. and A.M.d.R. Conceptualisation, S.M.; methodology, S.M., A.A. and A.M.d.R.; software, S.M. and V.A.; validation, S.M.; formal analysis, S.M., L.M.B. and V.A.; investigation, S.M.; resources, S.M. and A.M.d.R.; data curation, S.M. and A.A.; writing—original draft preparation, S.M. and L.M.B.; writing—review and editing, S.M., L.M.B. and V.A.; visualisation, S.M.; supervision, S.M., L.M.B., V.A.; A.A. and A.M.d.R.; project administration, S.M. All authors have read and agreed to the published version of the manuscript.

Funding: This research received no external funding.

Institutional Review Board Statement: The study was conducted according to the guidelines of the Declaration of Helsinki and approved by the Pharmacy and Therapeutics Committee of the Hospital Universitario Fundación de Alcorcón under use of drugs in special situations (Code reference TFGM2116).

Informed Consent Statement: Informed consent was obtained from all subjects involved in the study, as well as from the patients to publish this paper.

Data Availability Statement: Reported results can be found in the files of Centro de Investigaciones Biológicas Margarita Salas (CIB, CSIC) and in the files of Hospital Universitario Fundación Alcorcón (HUFA), Madrid, Spain.

Acknowledgments: We thank all patients for their help and the collaboration of Elia Pérez and all the research department of the University Hospital Alcorcón Foundation, which has helped us in the development of this work. We are also grateful to Belén Garzón and Laura García-Barrio from the CSIC, CTI (Technical Center of Informatics), for their help with statistics.

Conflicts of Interest: The authors declare no conflict of interest.

References

1. Garg, N.; Khunger, M.; Gupta, A.; Kumar, N. Optimal management of hereditary hemorrhagic telangiectasia. *J. Blood Med.* **2014**, *5*, 191–206.
2. Shovlin, C.L.; Guttmacher, A.E.; Buscarini, E.; Faughnan, M.E.; Hyland, R.H.; Westermann, C.J.J.; Kjeldsen, A.D.; Plauchu, H. Diagnostic criteria for Hereditary Hemorrhagic Telangiectasia (Rendu- Osler-Weber Syndrome). *Am. J. Med. Genet.* **2000**, *91*, 66–67. [CrossRef]
3. Faughnan, M.E.; Palda, V.A.; Garcia-Tsao, G.; Geisthoff, U.W.; McDonald, J.; Proctor, D.D.; Spears, J.; Brown, D.H.; Buscarini, E.; Chesnutt, M.S.; et al. International guidelines for the diagnosis and management of hereditary haemorrhagic telangiectasia. *J. Med. Genet.* **2011**, *48*, 73–87. [CrossRef]
4. Braverman, I.M.; Keh, A.; Jacobson, B.S. Ultrastructure and three-dimensional organization of the telangiectases of hereditary hemorrhagic telangiectasia. *J. Investig. Dermatol.* **1990**, *95*, 422–427. [CrossRef] [PubMed]
5. Aassar, O.S.; Friedman, C.M.; White, R.I. The Natural History of Epistaxis in Hereditary Hemorrhagic Telangiectasia. *Laryngoscope* **1991**, *101*, 977–980. [CrossRef] [PubMed]
6. Boyer, H.; Fernandes, P.; Le, C.; Yueh, B. Prospective randomized trial of sclerotherapy vs standard treatment for epistaxis due to hereditary hemorrhagic telangiectasia. *Int. Forum Allergy Rhinol.* **2015**, *5*, 435–440. [CrossRef] [PubMed]
7. Albiñana, V.; Cuesta, A.M.; Rojas, P.I.; Gallardo-Vara, E.; Recio-Poveda, L.; Bernabéu, C.; Botella, L.M. Review of Pharmacological Strategies with Repurposed Drugs for Hereditary Hemorrhagic Telangiectasia Related Bleeding. *J. Clin. Med.* **2020**, *9*, 1766. [CrossRef] [PubMed]
8. Morais, D.; Millás, T.; Zarrabeitia, R.; Botella, L.M.; Almaraz, A. Local sclerotherapy with polydocanol (Aethoxysklerol®) for the treatment of epistaxis in Rendu-Osler-Weber or hereditary hemorrhagic telangiectasia (HHT): 15 years of experience. *Rhinology* **2012**, *50*, 80–86. [CrossRef] [PubMed]
9. Esteban-Casado, S.; Martín de Rosales Cabrera, A.M.; Usarralde Pérez, A.; Martínez Simón, J.J.; Zhan Zhou, E.; Marcos Salazar, M.S.; Pérez Encinas, M.; Botella Cubells, L. Sclerotherapy and Topical Nasal Propranolol: An Effective and Safe Therapy for HHT-Epistaxis. *Laryngoscope* **2019**, *129*, 2216–2223. [CrossRef] [PubMed]
10. Zarrabeitia, R.; Señaris, B.; Rodríguez-Iglesias, J.; Megía, R.; Morales, C.; Marcos, S.; Fariñas-Álvarez, M.C.; Parra, J.A. Natural History of Epistaxis in a Spanish Population with Hereditary Haemorrhagic Telangiectasia (HHT). *Ann. Vasc. Med. Res.* **2016**, *3*, 1044.
11. Hoag, J.B.; Terry, P.; Mitchell, S.; Reh, D.; Merlo, C.A. An epistaxis severity score for hereditary hemorrhagic telangiectasia. *Laryngoscope* **2010**, *120*, 838–843. [CrossRef]
12. Herdman, M.; Badia, X.; Berra, S. EuroQol-5D: A simple alternative for measuring health-related quality of life in primary care. *Aten. Primaria* **2001**, *28*, 425–430. [CrossRef]
13. Yin, L.X.; Reh, D.D.; Hoag, J.B.; Mitchell, S.E.; Mathai, S.C.; Robinson, G.M.; Merlo, C.A. The minimal important difference of the epistaxis severity score in hereditary hemorrhagic telangiectasia. *Laryngoscope* **2016**, *126*, 1029–1032. [CrossRef]
14. Whitehead, K.J.; Sautter, N.B.; McWilliams, J.P.; Chakinala, M.M.; Merlo, C.A.; Johnson, M.H.; James, M.; Everett, E.M.; Clancy, M.S.; Faughnan, M.E.; et al. Effect of topical intranasal therapy on epistaxis frequency in patients with hereditary hemorrhagic telangiectasia: A randomized clinical trial. *JAMA* **2016**, *316*, 943–951. [CrossRef]
15. Zarrabeitia, R.; Fariñas-Álvarez, C.; Santibáñez, M.; Señaris, B.; Fontalba, A.; Botella, L.M.; Parra, J.A. Quality of life in patients with hereditary haemorrhagic telangiectasia (HHT). *Health Qual. Life Outcomes* **2017**, *15*, 19. [CrossRef]
16. Fang, J.; Chen, X.; Zhu, B.; Ye, H.; Zhang, W.; Guan, J.; Su, K. Thalidomide for Epistaxis in Patients with Hereditary Hemorrhagic Telangiectasia: A Preliminary Study. *Otolaryngol. Head Neck Surg.* **2017**, *157*, 217–221. [CrossRef]
17. Khoueir, N.; Borsik, M.; Camous, D.; Herman, P.; Verillaud, B. Injection of Bevacizumab and Cyanoacrylate for Hereditary Hemorrhagic Telangiectasia. *Laryngoscope* **2019**, *129*, 2210–2215. [CrossRef] [PubMed]

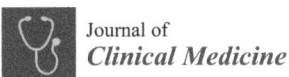

Article

Current Status of Clinical and Genetic Screening of Hereditary Hemorrhagic Telangiectasia Families in Hungary

Tamás Major [1,*], Zsuzsanna Bereczky [2,*], Réka Gindele [2], Gábor Balogh [2], Benedek Rácz [1,2], László Bora [3], Zsolt Kézsmárki [4], Boglárka Brúgós [5] and György Pfliegler [5]

1. Division of Otorhinolaryngology and Head & Neck Surgery, Kenézy Gyula Campus, University of Debrecen Medical Center, University of Debrecen, H-4031 Debrecen, Hungary; benedekrcz@gmail.com
2. Division of Clinical Laboratory Science, Department of Laboratory Medicine, Faculty of Medicine, University of Debrecen, H-4032 Debrecen, Hungary; gindele.reka@med.unideb.hu (R.G.); balogh.gabor@med.unideb.hu (G.B.)
3. Department of Radiology, Szent Lázár County Hospital, H-3100 Salgótarján, Hungary; crisicum@gmail.com
4. Division of Radiology, Kenézy Gyula Campus, University of Debrecen Medical Center, University of Debrecen, H-4031 Debrecen, Hungary; kezsmarki.zsolt@kenezy.unideb.hu
5. Division of Rare Diseases, Department of Internal Medicine Block B, Faculty of Medicine, University of Debrecen, H-4032 Debrecen, Hungary; brugosb@med.unideb.hu (B.B.); pfliegler@med.unideb.hu (G.P.)
* Correspondence: major.tamas@kenezy.unideb.hu (T.M.); zsbereczky@med.unideb.hu (Z.B.); Tel.: +36-52-511777 (ext. 1756) (T.M.); +36-52-431956 (Z.B.); Fax: +36-52-511755 (T.M.); +36-52-340011 (Z.B.)

Keywords: hereditary hemorrhagic telangiectasia; ENG; ACVRL1; SMAD4; germline mutation; genetic test; Curaçao criteria; family screening

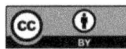

1. Introduction

Hereditary hemorrhagic telangiectasia (HHT) is a rare germline vascular malformation syndrome with a prevalence of 1:5000–1:10,000 [1,2]. HHT is listed in both the capillary (telangiectasia subgroup) and the arteriovenous malformation (AVM) groups in the 2018 classification from the International Society for the Study of Vascular Anomalies (ISSVA) [3]. Due to its complexity, HHT appears relatively late as a syndrome in medical history, starting with the fundamental papers of Rendu, Osler and Weber, published between 1896 and 1907 [2].

Telangiectases are mucocutaneous (1–2 mm in diameter), and AVMs are high-flow, solid organ arteriovenous shunts bypassing the intervening capillary bed [4]. Both telangiectases and AVMs show very characteristic localizations in HHT, reflected by the Curaçao criteria: 1. spontaneous, recurrent nosebleeds; 2. multiple telangiectases at characteristic sites (lips, oral cavity, fingers and nose); 3. visceral lesions such as gastrointestinal telangiectasia with or without bleeding including pulmonary, hepatic and cerebral AVMs (PAVMs, HAVMs and CAVMs, respectively); and 4. a first degree relative with HHT according to these criteria [5]. Major acute or chronic complications might be deduced through shunting (dyspnea, ischaemic strokes and brain abscesses by pulmonary right-to-left shunting, pulmonary hypertension and high output cardiac failure by left-to-right hepatic shunting, portal hypertension by hepatoportal shunting, encephalopathy by portohepatic shunting) and bleeding (hemorrhagic strokes, hemoptysis and anemia due to epistaxis or gastrointestinal bleeding) [6].

The majority of familial (germline) vascular malformations or syndromes including HHT are inherited in an autosomal-dominant trait with age-dependent penetrance, and mutations are usually family-specific [1]. Causative genes identified to date are ENG (encodes endoglin; mutations account for the HHT1 phenotype) [7] and ACVRL1 (encodes activin receptor-like kinase 1; mutations account for the HHT2 phenotype) [8] in 85% of

HHT families, SMAD4, accounting for the juvenile polyposis–HHT phenotype, in 2% of HHT families [9] and GDF2 (encodes bone morphogenic protein 9; mutations account for the extremely rare HHT5 phenotype) [10]. The phenotypic spectrum of HHT1 and HHT2 is slightly different, with an earlier onset of symptoms in HHT1, more PAVMs and CAVMs in HHT1 and more HAVMs in HHT2 [6], resulting in a generally more severe phenotype in HHT1. Each protein encoded by the above genes belongs to the transforming growth factor-beta (TGF-β) superfamily controlling angiogenesis. All variant types (missense, nonsense, splice-site, frameshift, in-frame deletions and insertions and finally, large deletions and insertions in 10% of cases) have been described throughout the ENG, ACVRL1 and SMAD4 [11]. On the other hand, the HHT Mutation Database on the Associated Regional and University Pathologists (ARUP) laboratory's website [12] enumerates 510 ENG and 572 ACVRL1 variants at present.

Being aware of the most frequently affected genes and their allele heterogeneity, the proposed molecular testing algorithm for HHT is ENG and ACVRL1 sequencing and a large deletion–insertion test (through multiplex ligation-dependent probe amplification, MLPA) followed by SMAD4 sequencing as well as MLPA if no variants of certain pathogenicity are found in the ENG and ACVRL1 genes [11,13].

The diagnosis of HHT remains a challenge, especially in probands. In a comprehensive study of 233 patients recruited between 2000 and 2009 [14], the diagnostic time lag (the interval between the first symptoms and the diagnosis of HHT) was 29.1 years for index cases and 22.6 years for non-index cases. Its first period was the interval between disease onset and the patient's referral to any physicians due to HHT-related manifestations (called the referral time lag), explained by the authors as being due to the poor knowledge of HHT in society. The long second period between the patients' referrals to a diagnosis of HHT is attributable to the unawareness of HHT within the medical community [14]. HHT is a rare disease with age-related penetrance of its multisystemic symptoms, and in addition, congenital PAVMs and CAVMs are most often asymptomatic until emerging as severe, acute complications in a subset of patients. The involved disciplines might address the symptoms one by one, often without the chance to assemble the underlying syndrome. At the University of Debrecen and the surrounding hospitals in Northeast Hungary, the management of HHT patients started a decade ago. The objective of this study is to give an account of the current status of the Hungarian HHT families' clinical and genetic screenings, performed in order to reduce the diagnostic time lag of the disease.

2. Patients and Methods

2.1. Patient Recruitment

The initial physical examinations were performed at the Division of Rare Diseases, Faculty of Medicine, University of Debrecen, in the Division of Otorhinolaryngology and Head and Neck Surgery, Kenézy Gyula Campus, University of Debrecen Medical Center; in the Department of Otorhinolaryngology, Ferenc Markhot County Hospital, Eger; and in the Department of Otolaryngology and Head and Neck Surgery, Borsod-Abaúj-Zemplén County Central Hospital and University Teaching Hospital, Miskolc, Hungary by the internist (G.P. and B.B.) and otorhinolaryngologist (T.M.) authors, respectively, all experts in HHT within their specialties. Patients with known or suspected HHT with habitation throughout Hungary presented themselves or were referred by their family doctors or specialists. The only well-defined denominator population involved in the study was the primary attendance area of the Ferenc Markhot County Hospital, Eger, Hungary (population of 225,339), where the stratified population screening of HHT was executed [15].

2.2. Clinical Evaluation

Our clinical HHT examination protocol started with a thorough medical history (nosebleeds, telangiectases, dyspnea, stroke, migraine, brain abscess, abdominal pain, anemia, hemoptysis, melena, etc. as well as family history concerning the same) as well as

ENT and internal (dyspnea, clubbing, hepatic bruits, etc.) physical examinations completed through the evaluation of each characteristic telangiectasis site.

Adult probands fulfilling at least 2 Curaçao criteria (mostly epistaxis, telangiectases or a first degree relative with HHT) underwent a visceral AVM screening through simultaneous non-enhanced and contrast-enhanced, arterial and venous phase chest and upper abdominal computed tomography (CT) (Siemens Somatom Definition AS 64; Siemens Shanghai Medical Equipment, Shanghai, China)) as well as a magnetic resonance (MR) examination (Siemens Magnetom Essenza 1.5 T; Siemens Shenzhen Magnetic Resonance, Shenzhen, China) of the brain following the "vascular malformation" protocol with T1 sagittal, T2 axial and T2 fluid-attenuated inversion recovery (FLAIR) coronal, diffusion-weighted imaging (DWI); susceptibility-weighted imaging (SWI); non-enhanced and contrast-enhanced 3D time-of-flight (TOF) angiography and postcontrast 3DT1 examinations. If patients underwent contrast-enhanced chest CT or brain MR with any other indications within three years prior to enrollment to our study, images were reassessed by the radiologists in our study group (L.B. and Z.K.) in order to reduce evaluation bias. Endoscopic examination of the upper or lower digestive tracts was offered at the suspicion of gastrointestinal bleeding or in the case of long-standing anemia disproportionate to epistaxis. Laboratory tests including complete blood count, iron status and liver function were recommended at the first visit. Pedigree charts were constructed using information from probands and senior family members. Proband evaluation was accomplished using genetic testing.

In pediatric patients under 18 years of age, a chest radiograph as well as pulse oximetry in supine (considered abnormal if SaO2 < 96%) and erect positions (abnormal if it decreased by $\geq 2\%$) was performed to screen for PAVMs. MR examination for CAVMs was offered to symptomatic children; otherwise, it was postponed until adulthood.

For at-risk family members, physical examinations were also performed. In the case of definite or suspected HHT, evaluations proceeded with the visceral AVM screening protocol. Genetic screening for the causative, family-specific mutation was offered for each at-risk family member, regardless of HHT status. If a family member's HHT status was clinically evaluated as "unlikely" but the family-specific mutation was detected (especially in younger individuals), the patient underwent the AVM screening.

2.3. Mutation Analysis

The isolation of genomic DNA from peripheral, citrated whole blood, and Sanger sequencing of the exons and flanking intronic sites of ENG, ACVRL1 and SMAD4 were performed as previously reported [16,17]. Three probands were tested using next-generation sequencing covering HHT causative genes (ACVRL1, ENG, SMAD4 and GDF2), among others [17].

In cases where no mutation was found through Sanger sequencing, MLPA analysis was performed using a SALSA MLPA Kit P093 HHT/HPAH (MRC-Holland, Amsterdam, The Netherlands). The MLPA data were analyzed using Coffalyser.Net Software (version 140721.1958, MRC-Holland, Amsterdam, The Netherlands, 2021).

2.4. Variant Assessment

Following screening for polymorphisms in the dbSNP and 1000 Genomes databases and in randomly selected, healthy control individuals ($n = 50$) from the framework of the Hungarian General Practitioners' Morbidity Sentinel Stations Program (HMSSP), representing the general Hungarian population [18], variants were verified in the Human Gene Mutation Database (HGMD) [19] and the Associated Regional and University Pathologist (ARUP) Mutation Database [12]. Novel variants were tested for familial cosegregation when several affected and non-affected at-risk family members were available. To assess the probability of the cosegregation of the variant with disease, the simplified method for cosegregation analysis (SISA) [20] was used. The pathogenicity of novel missense variants was assessed using Polyphen2 HumDiv and HumVar, MutPred2 and SIFT in silico prediction-modeling software and with the Franklin Genoox platform [21]. In the case of novel splice-site variants, the Human Splicing Finder software was used. Finally, variants were classified as pathogenic, likely pathogenic or variants of uncertain significance (VUS) on the basis of databases (known variants) or the standards and guidelines of the American College of Medical Genetics and Genomics (ACMG) [22].

2.5. The Algorithm of Cascade Family Screening

At-risk individuals awaiting screening in families with known mutations were classified as obligately or facultatively testable. The obligately testable family members were 1. first degree relatives of individuals positive for the family-specific mutation and 2. patients fulfilling ≥2 Curaçao criteria (suspected or definite HHT) and their first-degree relatives. The facultatively testable individuals were all asymptomatic first-degree relatives of individuals who tested positive in the obligate group (Figure 1).

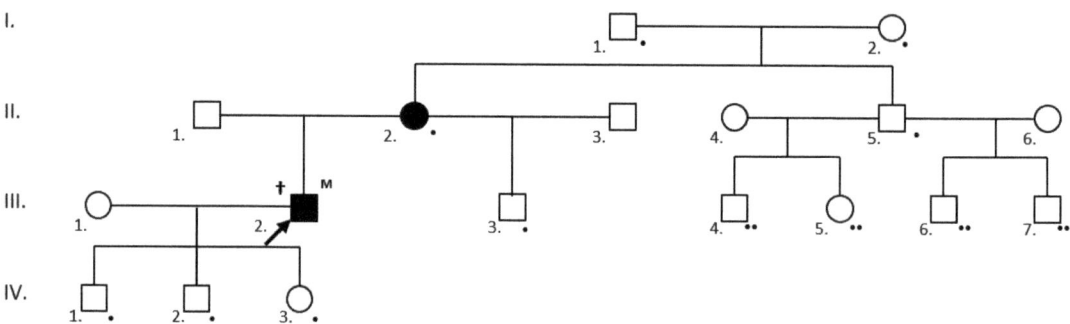

Figure 1. Cascade mutation screening in a family with a definite HHT (†) III.2. proband (arrow) with a novel, likely pathogenic ENG mutation (M). The following individuals were obligately testable (•): the IV.1., IV.2. and IV.3. first-degree asymptomatic relatives of the mutation carrier; the II.2. clinically affected first-degree relatives of the mutation carrier; and the III.3. (son), II.5. (sibling), I.1. and I.2. (parents) first-degree relatives of the affected II.2. individual. Individuals III.4., III.5., III.6 and III.7. became testable (facultatively testable at present) (••) if their father proved to be a mutation carrier at the obligate testing. Clinically and/or genetically affected individuals are shaded.

2.6. Statistical Analysis

The Kolmogorov–Smirnov test and Shapiro–Wilk test were performed to examine the normality of age distribution. Results regarding the continuous variable of age were expressed as mean ± SD. Between-group differences in age were analyzed using the Student's *t*-test. Differences in category frequencies were evaluated using the χ^2 test. A *p*-value of 0.05 or less was considered to indicate statistical significance. All statistical analyses were performed using the Statistical Package for the Social Sciences (SPSS 26.0), Chicago, IL, USA, 2021.

3. Results
3.1. Demographical Data

Including probands and at-risk family members, a total of 186 individuals of Hungarian ethnicity (84 males and 102 females) in 50 families (18 male and 32 female probands aged 56.5 ± 12.9 years; 66 male and 70 at-risk family members aged 35.8 ± 19.2 years) were evaluated for HHT using our clinical and genetic algorithm. One hundred and eighty-two members of the study cohort had a habitation in Hungary, with a predominance in the northeast at the time of the test (Figure 2a); the remainder were living in Austria, Germany, Great Britain and Italy. Probands' habitation (Figure 2b) followed a similar geographical distribution. In 24% of kindreds (12/50) only the probands were tested, while in 42% (21/50) 2–3 individuals, in 18% (9/50) 4–6 individuals, in 10% (5/50) 7–10 individuals and finally, in 6% (3/50) > 10 individuals were tested, giving a rate of 3.72 individuals/family.

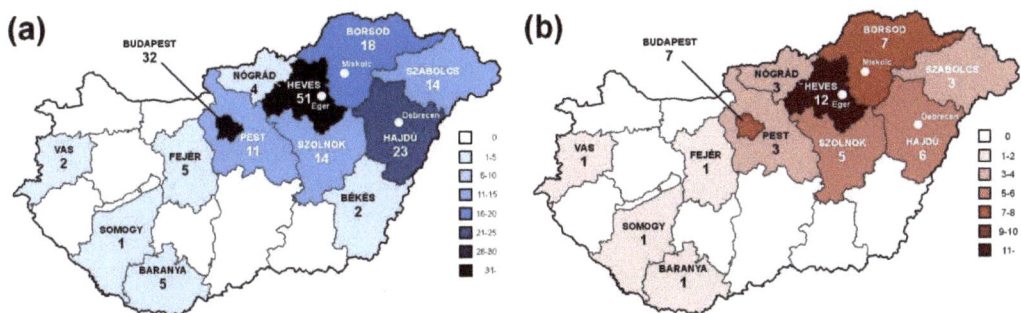

Figure 2. Distribution of all individuals (**a**) and probands (**b**) tested for HHT according to habitation in the 19 Hungarian counties as well as Budapest. The clinical and genetic HHT-testing institutions are indicated with white dots.

3.2. Mutation Analysis

A mutation was identified in 48 of the 50 families, giving a mutation detection rate of 96%. Eighteen different ENG mutations were detected in 53 individuals of 21 families (Figure 3). Fifteen variants were pathogenic or likely pathogenic, and 3 were VUS (the c.816+5G>A variant has a ≥99.22% probability of cosegregation by SISA). Thirteen of the ENG variants were published (3 of them by our study group) [23]. Splice-site and frameshift variants occurred most frequently. Two variants were each detected in two apparently unrelated families. The wild-type ENG allele was detected in 31 individuals.

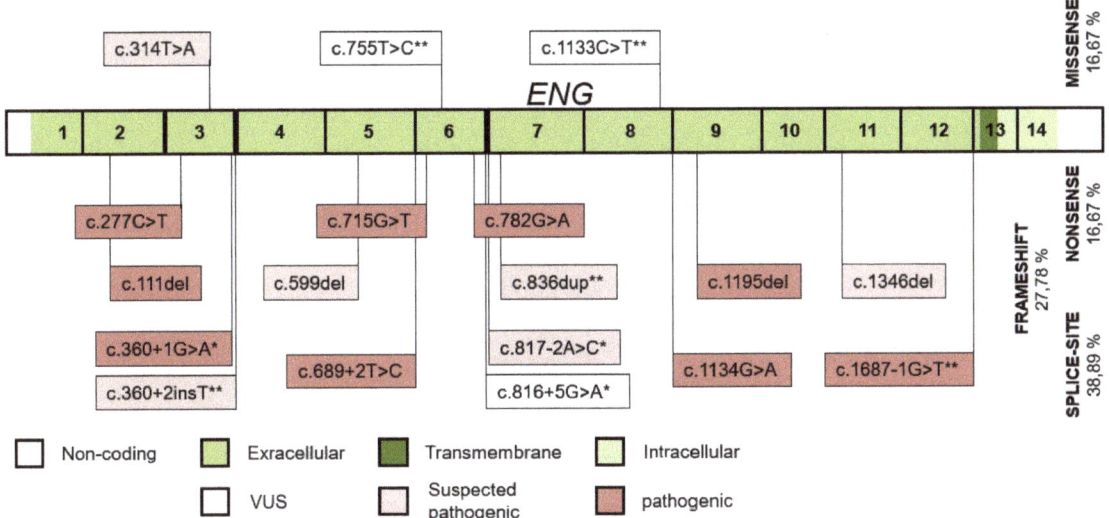

Figure 3. The distribution of ENG variants detected throughout the ENG exons and their intronic boundaries. Variants published by our study group and novel variants in this study are indicated with (*) and (**), respectively.

Sixteen ACVRL1 variants (Figure 4) were detected in 63 individuals of 26 kindreds, 10 of them were published (5 of them by our study group) [23]. Variants were pathogenic or likely pathogenic with the exception of 2 VUS. Three variants were shared by 2, 3 and 8 families. The predominant mutation type was missense. The wild-type ACVRL1 allele was detected in 34 individuals.

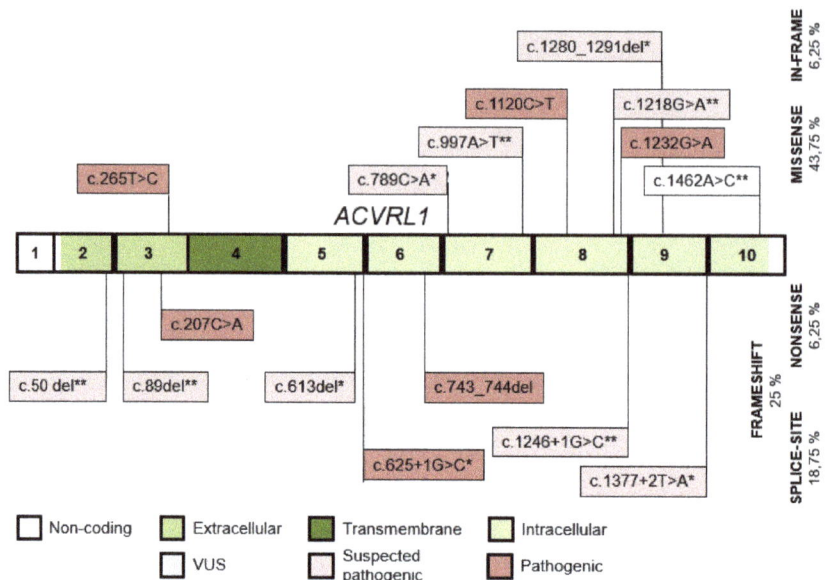

Figure 4. The distribution of ACVRL1 variants detected throughout the ACVRL1 exons and their intronic boundaries. Variants published by our study group and novel variants in this study are indicated with (*) and (**), respectively.

Thus, the ENG/ACVRL1 mutation rate was 1.13 (18/16) and the ENG/ACVRL1 family rate was 0.81 (21/26), while the ENG/ACVRL1 mutation positive individuals' rate was 0.84 (53/63).

A SMAD4 c.7A>G variant was identified in an additional kindred [17]. In the remaining two families (with 4 affected individuals) no mutation was detected despite performing the ENG, ACVRL1 and SMAD4 exon and flanking intronic sequencing and MLPA tests in the probands with definite HHT.

The hitherto unpublished variants and their evaluations of pathogenicity are detailed in Table 1.

Table 1. Novel ENG and ACVRL1 variants detected in this study.

Variant	Protein Change	Type	Population dbSNP 1000 Genomes HMSSP	Co-Segregation	SISA	In Silico Prediction Modeling Software	ACMG §
ENG							
c.360+2insT		SS	none	M: 1D		NA	LP
c.755T>C	p.Ile252Thr	MS	none	M: 2D		PolyPhen2 HumDiv *: possibly damaging PolyPhen2 HumVar *: probably damaging MutPred2 *: non-pathogenic/borderline SIFT **: affecting protein function	VUS
c.836dup	p.Cys279fs	FS	none	M: 1D		NA	LP
c.1133C>T	p.Ala378Val	MS	none	M: 1S I; w: 1NL		PolyPhen2 HumDiv *: possibly damaging PolyPhen2 HumVar *: benign MutPred2 *: non-pathogenic SIFT **: tolerated	VUS
c.1687-1G>T		SS	none	M: 3D + 1S PED	≥87.5%	NA	P

Table 1. Cont.

Variant	Protein Change	Type	Population dbSNP 1000 Genomes HMSSP	Co-Segregation	SISA	In Silico Prediction Modeling Software	ACMG §
ACVRL1							
c.50del #	p.Leu17Trpfs *2	FS	none			NA	LP
c.89del	p.Pro30Argfs *3	FS	none	M: 1S I		NA	LP
c.997A>T #	p.Ser333Cys	MS	none	M: 4D w: 1NL	≥87.5%	PolyPhen2 HumDiv *: probably damaging PolyPhen2 HumVar *: probably damaging MutPred2 *: likely pathogenic SIFT **: affecting protein function	LP
c.1218G>A #	p.Trp406 *	NS	none	M: 2D w: 2NL		NA	LP
c.1246+1G>C #		SS	none	M: 1D + 1NL I; w: 2NL		NA	LP
c.1462A>C	p.Thr488Pro	MS	none	M: 2D + 1S PED		PolyPhen2 HumDiv *: probably damaging PolyPhen2 HumVar *: probably damaging MutPred2 *: likely pathogenic SIFT **: affecting protein function	VUS

Abbreviations and legend: Under Variant, (#), the specific nucleotides affected in the novel variant are also targets of different, previously described HHT variants [12]. Under variant type (Type), FS: frameshift; MS: missense; NS: nonsense; SS: splice-site. Under Cosegregation, D: clinically definite HHT; (I): incomplete clinical evaluation; M: family-specific mutation; NL: HHT clinically not likely; (PED): pediatric patient; S: clinically suspected HHT; w: wild-type ENG/ACVRL1 allele. Under In Silico Prediction Modeling Software, (*): pathogenic with a score > 0.5; (**): pathogenic with a score < 0.05; NA: not applicable. Under ACMG, (§): pathogenicity was predicted using the Franklin Genoox platform [21]. LP: likely pathogenic; P: pathogenic.

3.3. Genotype–Phenotype Correlations

Patient numbers and gender rates in the overall ($n = 116$) HHT1 + HHT2 cohorts and within their subdivisions based upon their fulfilled Curaçao criteria are shown in Table 2. Interestingly, in the definite HHT subgroup, the number of females was significantly higher among HHT2 compared to HHT1 patients ($p = 0.020$). This difference remained significant concerning the overall HHT2 vs HHT1 cohorts ($p = 0.040$). Five asymptomatic individuals (0–33 years of age) carried the family-specific ACVRL1 mutation. In addition, in 31 (12 males and 19 females, aged 35.6 ± 18.3 years) and 34 (17 males and 17 females, aged 35.1 ± 21.5 years) unaffected individuals of the HHT1 and HHT2 kindreds, respectively, the wild-type ENG and ACVRL1 alleles were detected.

Table 2. Demographical data of the HHT1 and HHT2 cohorts.

	HHT1	HHT2	HHT1+HHT2
Overall			
No. (male/female)	53 (31/22)	63 (24/39)	116 (55/61)
Age (years) ± SD	46.1 ± 18.0	43.5 ± 19.9	44.7 ± 19.1
3 or 4 clinical criteria exist			
No. (male/female)	44 (24/20)	47 (14/33)	91 (38/53)
Age (years) ± SD	49.2 ± 16.4	50.0 ± 15.7	49.6 ± 16.1
2 clinical criteria exist			
No. (male/female)	9 (7/2)	11 (7/4)	20 (14/6)
Age (years) ± SD	31.1 ± 17.8	30.0 ± 18.1	30.5 ± 18.0
1 clinical criterion exists			
No. (male/female)	0	5 (3/2)	5 (3/2)
Age (years) ± SD		12.0 ± 11.6	12.0 ± 11.6

Patient age refers to the age at enrollment to our study.

All probands and at-risk family members underwent the ENT and internal physical examination protocols. However, the visceral AVM screening was incomplete at the time of writing the manuscript in a subset of patients, while others refused the imaging studies. The results of the clinical evaluations are shown in Table 3.

Table 3. Clinical manifestations in the HHT1 and HHT2 cohorts based on the Curaçao criteria.

	HHT1	HHT2	p Value	HHT1 + HHT2
Epistaxis				
Overall	53/53 (100%)	55/63 (87.3%)	0.007	108/116 (93.1%)
Definite	44/44 (100%)	46/47 (97.9%)	NS	90/91 (98.9%)
Suspected	9/9 (100%)	9/11 (81.8%)	NS	18/20 (90%)
Telangiectasia				
Overall	33/53 (62.3%)	48/63 (76.2%)	NS	81/116 (69.8%)
Definite	33/44 (75%)	46/47 (97.9%)	0.001	79/91 (86.8%)
Suspected	0/9 (0%)	2/11 (18.2%)	NS	2/20 (10%)
PAVM overall [1]	22/41 (53.7%) [2]	2/46 (4.3%) [2]	<0.001	24/87 (27.6%) [2]
CAVM overall [3]	4/21 (19.0%) [2]	1/36 (2.8%) [2]	NS	5/57 (8.8%) [2]
HAVM overall [3]	7/29 (24.1%) [2]	19/39 (48.7%) [2]	0.047	26/68 (38.2%) [2]
GI telangiectasia [4]	9/53 (17.0%)	7/63 (11.1%) [2]	NS	16/116 (13.8%) [2]

Legend: [1]: PAVM screening was offered to all pediatric and adult patients with mutations and/or fulfilling ≥ 2 diagnostic criteria; [2] Only individuals undergoing the screening protocol of the particular visceral organ constitute the denominators; [3]: CAVM and HAVM screenings were offered to adults only; [4] Endoscopic evaluations of upper and/or lower gastrointestinal mucosal telangiectases were performed as needed (see Section 2.2); NS: non-significant.

Epistaxis was observed in all-but-one definite HHT1 + HHT2 patients. The exception was a 34-year-old HHT2 female with mucocutaneous telangiectases at characteristic sites, HAVM and a positive family history. Nosebleeds were significantly more common in the overall HHT1 cohort. Telangiectasia was more common in HHT2 patients in the overall HHT cohort, and this difference was significant in the definite subgroup. In the suspected HHT subgroup, all patients had epistaxis (90%) or telangiectasia (10%) as the second criterion added to their family histories.

Concerning visceral lesions, PAVMs were significantly more common in the HHT1 group. Four patients (3 with HHT1 and 1 with HHT2) had cerebral abscess. A HHT2 patient died of this at the age of 42 years. He had recurrent nosebleeds and mucocutaneous telangiectases, but he was not tested for HHT when alive. One year prior to his death, he was diagnosed with polycythemia (hemoglobin 20.6 g/dL) and tested for the JAK2 V617F variant with a negative result. A chest radiogram did not show any soft-tissue opacities, but CT was not performed. No pulmonary masses were described in his autopsy report. As the family-specific ACVRL1 c.50del was detected in his mother (proband with definite HHT) and daughter (with suspected HHT) six years later, his preserved DNA was also screened for this variant, and the mutation was detected. The three HHT1 patients with cerebral abscess had a detectable causative PAVM (Figure 5a,b) and in two of them, the cerebral abscess preceded the diagnosis of PAVM. The third HHT1 patient was a 22-year-old male with clubbing, dyspnea on exertion, polycythemia and a large pulmonary soft-tissue mass at onset, resulting in a long-term differential diagnostic pitfall [24]. In summary, the prevalence of cerebral abscess in the cohort with unambiguous PAVM and the overall HHT1 + HHT2 cohorts was 12.5% (3/24) and 3.4% (4/116), respectively.

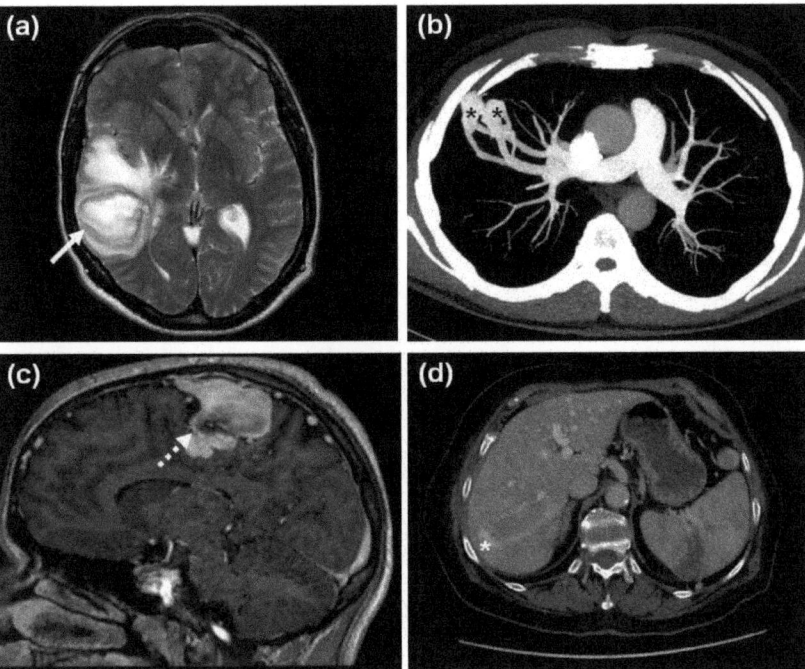

Figure 5. Visceral manifestations of HHT. (**a**) An axial plane, T2-weighted MR image of a cerebral abscess (white arrow) in the right temporal lobe of a 43-year-old HHT1 male and (**b**) the axial plane maximum intensity projection (MIP) CT image of the underlying 20 mm and 16 mm PAVMs (black asterisks) and their feeding vessels in the periphery of the right S3 segment in the same patient; (**c**) A 3DT1 postcontrast sagittal plane image of a CAVM (white dotted arrow) in the right parietal lobe of a 21-year-old male with HHT1; (**d**) An axial plane venous phase CT image showing a curved portovenous HAVM (white asterisk) with feeding vessels in the right liver lobe of a 73-year-old female HHT2 patient.

CAVMs were shown in 8.8% of all HHT patients undergoing brain MR with a near significant ($p = 0.056$) predominance in HHT1. Three of them were asymptomatic, and one had a chronic headache (Figure 5c). HAVMs (Figure 5d) were significantly more common in HHT2. Neither physical signs (bruits, palpable masses) nor comorbidities (portal hypertension, high output cardiac failure, hepatic encephalopathy, etc.) unambiguously associated with HAVMs were observed. Symptomatic gastrointestinal telangiectases were detected in 13.8% of the overall HHT cohort, with a mild HHT1 predominance.

Within our HHT1 + HHT2 cohort, 24 individuals were minors. Their results are detailed in Table 4. Among the 9 patients with pathogenic or likely pathogenic variants, the leading symptom was epistaxis in 5 cases, followed by telangiectases in 2 cases. Considering visceral lesions, only PAVM screening was performed with negative results; otherwise, no patients were found with history or symptoms suggesting cerebral or hepatic AVMs. Fifteen individuals showed the wild-type ENG and ACVRL1 alleles.

Table 4. Clinical and genetic data of pediatric patients.

Kindreds	Male	Female
HHT1 family members (*n* = 8)		
Individuals with ENG mutation		
3 or 4 clinical criteria exist	-	-
2 clinical criteria exist	12y (E); 13y (E)	-
1 clinical criterion exists	-	-
Wild-type individuals	4y, 11y, 12y	6y, 7y, 17y
HHT2 family members (*n* = 16)		
Individuals with ACVRL1 mutation		
3 or 4 clinical criteria exist	-	9y (E,T)
2 clinical criteria exist	1y (E), 11y (T)	15y (E)
1 clinical criterion exists	0y, 4y	3y
Wild-type individual	5y, 7y, 8y, 11y, 13y	1y, 11y, 11y, 14y

Legend: y: years of age; E: epistaxis; T: telangiectasia.

A novel SMAD4 c.7A>G variant classified as a VUS was found in a 64-year-old female. She had recurrent nosebleeds, oral and lower lip telangiectases and two first-degree relatives with epistaxis. Neither the patient nor the kindred had a history of JPS, gastric or colon cancers. She had no anemia. Endoscopic examinations of the upper and lower gastrointestinal tract were offered, but she refused these. Her family was unavailable for clinical and genetic screening as well. On the basis of her incomplete evaluation, we could not determine whether she had a pure HHT or a JP–HHT phenotype.

3.4. Cascade Family Screening

Pedigree charts were constructed in 32 kindreds with 23 ENG/ACVRL1 variants (20 of them pathogenic or likely pathogenic in addition to 3 VUS). Table 5 shows the momentary states of the cascade mutation screening. The HHT mutation status was clarified in 156 individuals, 24 refused testing, an additional 151 were obligately testable, and 26 were facultatively testable.

Table 5. Cascade mutation screening: results and future tasks.

Gene	Variant	M+			w	Non-Testable	Refused Screening	Obligately Testable	Facultatively Testable
		≥3 1	2 1	1 1					
ENG	c.111del	1	0	0	2	0	0	0	0
	c.314T>A	1	0	0	1	0	0	2	0
	c.360+1G>A	3	0	0	8	0	1	0	0
	c.816+5G>A §	6	2	0	6	0	7	5	0
	c.817-2A>C (2)	11	1	0	10	0	7	7	0
	c.1134G>A	1	1	0	0	0	0	2	0
	c.1195del	1	0	0	0	0	0	12	2
	c.1346del	1	0	0	1	0	0	2	2
	c.1687-1G>T	1	1	0	0	0	5	0	0

Table 5. Cont.

Gene	Variant	M+			w	Non-Testable	Refused Screening	Obligately Testable	Facultatively Testable
		≥3 1	2 1	1 1					
ACVRL1	c.50del	3	1	0	0	0	0	2	2
	c.207C>A	1	0	0	6	7	0	3	0
	c.265T>C (3)	3	0	0	0	0	0	41	3
	c.613del	1	0	0	1	0	0	3	0
	c.625+1G>C (6)	16	4	3	14	2	3	6	0
	c.743_744del	1	0	0	0	0	0	8	0
	c.789C>A	1	1	1	0	0	0	3	0
	c.997A>T	4	0	0	1	1	0	17	7
	c.1120C>T	3	0	0	0	0	0	13	1
	c.1218G>A	2	0	0	2	0	0	2	0
	c.1232G>A	2	0	0	2	0	0	3	3
	c.1246+1G>C	2	0	0	2	0	0	6	4
	c.1280_1291del	1	1	0	0	0	0	8	2
	c.1377+2T>A (2)	3	1	0	4	0	1	6	0
	Total:	69	13	4	60	10	24	151	26
	Screening status	156 clarified					24 refuses	177 testable	

Abbreviations and legend: Under Variant, (§) is a VUS with a ≥ 99.22% probability of cosegregation by SISA; all other variants are pathogenic or likely pathogenic under ACMG Guidelines; the number of kindreds with the same variant is shown in brackets. M: individuals with the family-specific mutation; 1: the number of fulfilled clinical criteria; w: individuals with the wild-type ENG/ACVRL1 alleles. "Non-testable": the descendants of wild-type individuals in HHT families. "Obligately" or "Facultatively" testable: See Section 2.5 for legends.

4. Discussion

At present, we have 186 clinically and genetically tested individuals from 50 families (with provenience to the northeast in the majority of cases) at our HHT Centre in Debrecen, Hungary, corresponding to an individual/family rate of 3.72 and a patient/family rate of 2.42. These data are comparable with other studies evaluating a minimum of 100 HHT patients, ranging from 3.74 to 4.52 and 2.08 to 4.93, respectively (Table 6). In accordance with an autosomal dominant disease, the male-to-female rate in the overall HHT cohort was approximately equal (55/63). The only exception was the definite HHT2 cohort, in which a pronounced female predominance was observed (male-to-female rate of 19/33). Several studies report a female preponderance among patients diagnosed with HHT [25,26] as well as among patients identified through the analysis of HHT medical codes from a computerized general practice database yielding a representative sample of the UK population [27] or through combinations strongly suggestive of HHT in a US health insurance database [28]. This gender bias has been explained through behavioral factors (wider access of women to healthcare resources needed due to contraception, pregnancy and childcare) and biological factors [27].

Table 6. Comparison of the genetic results of some HHT studies evaluating a minimum of 100 patients.

Reference	Population [1] HHT Centre [2]	Molecular Analysis	Probands with Mutations/Total	ENG/ACVRL1 Mutation Rate	ENG/ACVRL1 Family Rate	ENG/ACVRL1 Pt Rate	Pts/Family [3] Inds/Family [4]
[4]	Utah, US [2]	ENG/ACVRL1 SS	26/34 (76.5%)	14/10 (1.4)	14/12 (1.17)	61/50 (1.22)	111/26 (4.27) [3]
[29]	Multicentric (US, Australia, Canada, Japan) [2]	ENG/ACVRL1 SS + 5′UTR SS + LDI	137/200 (68.5%)	71/42 (1.69)	77/50 (1.54)	ND	ND
[30]	Norwegian national study [1]	ENG/ACVRL1/ SMAD4 SS + LDI	total: 105/113 (92.9%) LP+P: 97/113 (85.8%)	total: 30/27 (1.11) LP+P: 30/23 (1.30) SMAD4: 0	total: 42/63 (0.67) LP+P: 39/58 (0.67)	ND	237/97 (2.44) 3 423/113 (3.74) 4
[31,32]	French HHT network [1]	ENG/ACVRL1 SS + 5′UTR SS + LDI, SMAD4 SS	D: 119/136 (87.5%)	D: 42/56 (0.75) SMAD4: 0	D: 40/79 (0.51)		
[25]	French–Italian HHT network [1]					91/250 (0.36)	343/135 (2.54) 3
[33]	Bari, Italy [2]						135/65 (2.08) [3]
[34]	Utrecht, The Netherlands [2]	ENG/ACVRL1 SS + LDI	97/104 (93.3%)	40/31 (1.29)	55/42 (1.31)		
[35]					63/40 (1.58)		508/103 (4.93) 3
[36]	Pavia-Crema, Italy [2]	ENG/ACVRL1 SS	101/137 (73.7%)	26/50 (0.52)	29/72 (0.40)		263/101 (2.60) 3 457/101 (4.52) 4
[37]	Spanish RiHHTa registry [1]	ENG/ACVRL1/ SMAD4 SS, NGS + LDI		16/25 (0.64)		36/77 (0.47)	
[13]	Danish national study [1]	ENG/ACVRL1/ SMAD4 SS + LDI	95/107 (88.8%)	29/32 (0.91) SMAD4: 3 fam	47/45 (1.04) SMAD4: 3 fam	151/132 (1.14) SMAD4: 5 pts	320/107 (3.06) 3
This study	Debrecen, Hungary [2]	ENG/ACVRL1/ SMAD4 SS, NGS + LDI	48/50 (96%)	18/16 (1.13) SMAD4: 1 fam	21/26 (0.81) SMAD4: 1 fam	53/63 (0.84) SMAD4: 1 pt	121/50 (2.42) [3] 186/50 (3.72) [4]

Abbreviations: [1]: study population defined; [2]: HHT center-defined; [3]: patients/family rate; [4]: individuals/family rate; D: definite HHT; fam: family; ind: individual; LDI: large deletion/insertion testing; LP: likely pathogenic variant; ND: not detailed; NGS: next-generation sequencing; P: pathogenic variant; pt: patient; SS: Sanger sequencing; 5′UTR: 5′ untranslated region.

All of the above HHT studies and the vast majority of papers in the literature are from Europe or North America, resulting in a publication bias. The methods of ENG, ACVRL1 and SMAD4 variant detection differ, and in particular, earlier studies lacked large deletion/insertion [4,36] or SMAD4 testing [4,29,36], accounting for approximately 10% and 2% of all HHT mutations, respectively [11]. In addition, the mutation detection rate is affected by the proband selection for the test, too. The strict application of the Curaçao criteria in probands (i.e., fulfillment of at least 3 criteria) resulted in an ENG and ACVRL1 mutation detection rate of 96.1% in a recent study [38], matching ours. Among our probands, only four were evaluated as having suspected HHT, but their AVM screenings were incomplete. All of them had a likely pathogenic ENG or ACVRL1 variant. The other 48 probands (including the 2 without detectable mutations) were definite HHT patients.

The "ENG/ACVRL1 rate" affecting HHT phenotype in a population is often described with some inaccuracy in the literature. In our opinion, this rate consists of three components: First, the ENG/ACVRL1 mutation rate shows considerable variation in different populations ranging from 0.52 to 1.69, even in larger cohorts (Table 6). This rate reflects the real allele heterogeneity of a given population, distorted by a potential referral bias associated with the HHT phenotype [35]. Second, in addition to this referral bias, the ENG/ACVRL1 proband (family) rate (ranging from 0.40 to 1.58) is further distorted by founder effects [39]. Three ACVRL1 founder variants detected in 24, 7 and 5 families accounted for 37.1% (36/97) of all mutation-positive kindreds in the Norwegian national HHT study [30]. The French founder variant (ACVRL1 c.1112_1113dupG) was detected in 17% (17/100) of families in the French HHT network [31]; four years later, 35 families were known to have this variant [40]. The Danish founder (ENG c.360C>A) accounted for 13.7% (13/95) of all family-specific variants in a national study [13]. In each of the above variants, the founder effect was confirmed by haplotype analysis. Third, the ENG/ACVRL1 patient rate might be further biased by the efficacy of family screening. In our experience, large kindreds living in relatively closed communities (e.g., the ENG c.817-2A>C kindred with 22 individuals in our study, the majority of them living in the same village) or kindreds with more severely affected individuals (e.g., two cerebral abscesses and a bleeding PAVM in the ENG c.816+5G>A kindred) show more willingness to participate in the family screening.

Demonstrating the ENG/ACVRL1 rate, the Hungarian founder ACVRL1 c.625 + 1G > C variant, 1 of the 34 unique ENG and ACVRL1 variants in our study, accounted for 16.7% (8/48) of the HHT1 + HHT2 kindreds and 23.3% (27/116) of the HHT1 + HHT2 patients at the time of the study.

In our ENG cohort, three variants were found in two families each. The ENG c.817-2A > C families share common ancestors detected by genealogical testing [39], the ENG c.1346del families live 20 km apart, and the ENG c.1687-1G>T kindreds have a shared, otherwise-rare surname. In the ACVRL1 cohort, beyond the above c.625+1G>C founder variant, the c.265T>C and c.1377+2T>A variants were shared by three and two unrelated probands, respectively, originating from neighboring villages in both cases.

The type and intragenic distribution of the ENG and ACVRL1 variants correspond with literature data, with their missense predominance and their predilection to exons 3 and 8 in ACVRL1, and even distribution of variants throughout the extracellular exons, with less missense variants in ENG [4,12,36].

Epistaxis and telangiectasia are, by far, the most frequent clinical manifestations of HHT, with age-related penetrance of both [4,25,41]. Our data confirm this through the epistaxis and telangiectasia prevalence of 93.1% and 76.2% in the overall cohort, respectively. The age-related penetrance is shown by a higher prevalence of the two criteria in the definite compared to the suspected cohorts in both HHT1 and HHT2. The onset of epistaxis precedes telangiectasia [2,41]. Although the onset of symptoms was not assessed in our study, in suspected HHT patients (aged 30.5 years) fulfilling family history plus another criterion, epistaxis was recorded in 90% and telangiectasia in the remaining 10% of cases.

Concerning the overall HHT1 and HHT2 groups, epistaxis was significantly more common in the HHT1 group. The number of asymptomatic mutation carriers in the two groups (0 HHT1 versus 5 HHT2) might account for this difference. In contrast, telangiectasia was significantly less frequent in definite HHT1 compared with HHT2. The age-related onset of symptoms might be the explanation for this [25,41]. In young adults, the coexistence of epistaxis (with earlier onset than in telangiectasia), a congenital AVM and family history is sufficient for categorization as definite HHT. Indeed, when reviewing the fulfilment of clinical criteria, 6 definite HHT1 patients aged 22–37 years were found with epistaxis, PAVM and family history, all lacking telangiectasia for the present.

Our visceral AVM screening protocol corresponds to the international HHT guidelines [42,43]. CT as a PAVM screening method is approved by the HHT guidelines in centers without expertise in transthoracic contrast echocardiography (TTCE) [42]. CT screening of HAVM is also regarded as appropriate in HHT guidelines [42], and furthermore, PAVM and HAVM screenings can be performed simultaneously in this way.

The visceral manifestations observed in our study were compared with others enrolling a minimum of 100 patients. Although the study cohorts (all patients versus adults only), the methodology and the indications (all patients versus symptomatic) of visceral screenings were rather different, PAVMs and CAVMs were significantly more prevalent in HHT1, while HAVMs had a predominance in HHT2 (Table 7). Our results are in accordance with the literature in the case of all three types of visceral AVMs. The prevalence of cerebral abscesses in the PAVM (12.5%) and the overall HHT1 + HHT2 cohorts (3.4%) also corresponds with reported data [44,45]. Gastrointestinal telangiectases show a wide range of overall prevalence in HHT, depending on the indication rather than on the methodology of screening; the majority of these lesions are asymptomatic [46,47]. Symptomatic lesions occur in 11–22% of HHT cases, with non-significant prevalence differences between HHT1 and HHT2 [4,13,37].

Table 7. Clinical manifestations of HHT1 and HHT2 in studies evaluating a minimum of 100 patients.

Ref.	Cohort	PAVM		CAVM		HAVM		GI Lesion	
		HHT1	HHT2	HHT1	HHT2	HHT1	HHT2	HHT1	HHT2
[4]	Utah, US [2]	36/61 (59%) $p = 0.002$	13/45 (28.9%)	10/61 (16.4%) $p = 0.012$	1/50 (2%)	1/59 (1.7%) $p < 0.001$	13/47 (27.7%)	7/39 (18%) bleeding	8/39 (21%) bleeding
[29]	Multicentric (US, Australia, Canada, Japan) [2]	52/77 (67.5%)	24/50 (48%)	7/77 (9.1%)	0	2/77 (2.6%)	7/50 (14%)	7/77 (9.1%)	5/50 (10%)
[25]	French–Italian HHT network [1]	sy: 32/93 (34.4%) $p < 0.001$ asy: 27/50 (54%) $p < 0.0001$	sy: 13/250 (5.2%) asy: 19/149 (12.8%)	sy: 2/93 (2.2%) NS asy: 2/22 (9.1%) NS	sy: 3/250 (1.2%) asy: 2/50 (4%)	sy: 0 NS asy: 20/46 (43.5%) NS	sy: 19/250 (7.6%) asy: 87/151 (57.6%)	6/93 (6.5%) $p = 0.017$	41/250 (16.4%)
[33]	Bari, Italy [2]	34/45 (75.5%) $p < 0.0005$ Large #: 21/34 (61.8%) $p < 0.0001$	34/77 (44.1%) Large #: 6/34 (17.6%)	9/43 (20.9%) $p < 0.0002$	0	27/45 (60%) $p < 0.01$	64/77 (83.1%)	18/30 (60%) NS	24/47 (51.1%)
[35]	Utrecht, The Netherlands [2]	167/343 (48.7%) $p = 1.2 \times 10^{-16}$	6/114 (5.3%)	38/260 (14.6%) $p = 0.0015$	1/76 (1.3%)	11/144 (7.6%) $p = 8.7 \times 10^{-7}$	13/32 (40.6%)	56/78 (71.8%) NS	19/29 (65.5%)
[37]	Spanish RiHHTa registry [1]	20/36 (55.5%) $p < 0.005$	11/77 (14.3%)	3/36 (8.3%) $p < 0.005$	1/77 (1.3%)	9/36 (25%) NS, $p = 0.075$	33/77 (42.8%)	Upper: 8/36 (22.2%) NS Lower: 3/36 (8.3%)	9/77 (11.7%) 3/77 (3.9%)
[13]	Danish national study [1]	79/151 (52.3%) $p < 0.001$	17/132 (12.9%)	2/16 (25%)	1/7 (14.3%)	2/5 (40%)	8/11 (72.7%)	28/151 (18.5%) NS	15/132 (11.4%)
This study	Debrecen, Hungary [2]	22/41 (53.7%) $p < 0.001$	2/46 (4.3%)	4/21 (19.0%) NS, $p = 0.056$	1/36 (2.8%)	7/29 (24.1%) $p = 0.047$	19/39 (48.7%)	9/53 (17%) NS	7/63 (11.1%)

Abbreviations: [1]: study population-defined; [2]: HHT center-defined; (#): A large PAVM is defined as a lesion > 3 mm [33]; asy: asymptomatic; NS: non-significant; sy: symptomatic.

A total of 24 pediatric individuals were tested; the family-specific ENG or ACVRL1 variant was detected in 9 of them. Three patients, with a newborn among them (mean age of 2.3 years), were asymptomatic, 5 (aged 10.4 years) had suspected HHT (4 with epistaxis and 1 with telangiectasia plus family history), and the only definite HHT patient was a 12-year-old female. None of them showed symptoms suggestive of visceral lesions. On the other hand, in contrast to the 2011 international HHT guidelines [42] and their 2020 amendments [43], CAVMs were not screened through MR, and the PAVM screening method lacked TTCE. Pediatric CAVM screening is a controversial point in the literature, as it requires sedation or anesthesia [43], the prevalence of CAVMs is relatively low (corresponding with the adulthood CAVM prevalence), and only a subset of them are treated [48]. Thus, in some HHT centers, including ours, screening of asymptomatic individuals for CAVMs is postponed until adulthood [49]. With awareness of the prevalence of congenital

HHT visceral lesions, it is conceivable that PAVMs or CAVMs will be detected in a subset of our pediatric patients through the AVM screening at 18 years of age.

The 5 asymptomatic pediatric mutation carriers were phenotypically indistinguishable from the 15 children with wild-type alleles. The confirmation or exclusion of disease in young asymptomatic family members is the main indication for genetic testing in HHT.

Thorough clinical and genetic family screening can reduce the diagnostic time lag in at-risk individuals. In order to do this, a cascade family screening has been developed. Pedigree charts have been constructed for 32 of the 48 kindreds with known variants. The 32 probands have yielded 148 tested and 151 obligately testable at-risk individuals so far. Thus, HHT status is clarified in 180 individuals at present, 24 of whom (13.3%) refused clinical and genetic testing. The cohort of non-testable individuals ($n = 10$) might be somewhat larger, as descendants of wild-type individuals were removed from the pedigree charts in the first years of the study. Furthermore, identification of novel branches on the pedigrees is expected to continually widen the testable cohort.

The main limitation of our study is the incomplete AVM screening in a subset of patients. CAVMs are not screened in childhood, and childhood PAVM screening differs from that of adulthood. TTCE needs to be started in our institution as the first-line PAVM screening method in both children and adults. In addition, a subset of mutation carriers did not give their consent for the visceral AVM screening. Finally, the COVID-19 pandemic, exerting an extreme burden on the Hungarian healthcare system, also hindered the imaging evaluation in a minority of patients.

5. Conclusions

We provide the first comprehensive HHT study from Eastern Europe, evaluating 186 individuals from 50 HHT families. Considering the ENG/ACVRL1 variant, family and patient rates and in addition, the distribution of symptoms in HHT1 and HHT2, the genetic and clinical properties of our Hungarian HHT cohort were comparable with literature data. Eleven novel variants were found (5 in the ENG and 6 in the ACVRL1 genes). Both the pitfalls of diagnosing HHT in probands and the significance of a thorough family screening are emphasized in order to reduce the diagnostic time lag in at-risk individuals.

Author Contributions: Conceptualization, T.M., Z.B. and G.P.; methodology, T.M., G.P., B.B., R.G.; L.B. and Z.K.; software, G.B. and B.R.; validation, Z.B.; investigation, T.M., G.P., B.B. and R.G.; resources, Z.B.; writing—original draft preparation, T.M.; writing—review and editing, Z.B. and G.P.; funding acquisition, Z.B. All authors have read and agreed to the published version of the manuscript.

Funding: This research was funded by the European Union under European Regional Development Fund, grant number GINOP-2.3.2-15-2016-00039 and by the National Research, Development and Innovation Office, Hungarian Ministry of Innovation and Technology, grant numbers OTKA K116228 and K139293. The APC was funded by the University of Debrecen.

Institutional Review Board Statement: The study was conducted according to the guidelines of the Declaration of Helsinki and approved by the Committee of the Hungarian Scientific Council on Health (protocol code 28676-7/2017/EÜIG).

Informed Consent Statement: Informed consent was obtained from all subjects involved in the study.

Data Availability Statement: The data presented in this study are available on request from the corresponding author. The data are not publicly available due to privacy and ethical considerations.

Conflicts of Interest: The authors declare no conflict of interest.

References

1. Borst, A.J.; Nakano, T.A.; Blei, F.; Adams, D.M.; Duis, J. A primer on a comprehensive genetic approach to vascular anomalies. *Front. Pediatr.* **2020**, *8*, 579591. [CrossRef]
2. Sharathkumar, A.A.; Shapiro, A. Hereditary haemorrhagic telangiectasia. *Haemophilia* **2008**, *14*, 1269–1280. [CrossRef]
3. ISSVA Classification for Vascular Anomalies. Available online: https://www.issva.org/UserFiles/file/ISSVA-Classification-2018.pdf (accessed on 5 June 2021).

4. Bayrak-Toydemir, P.; McDonald, J.; Markewitz, B.; Lewin, S.; Miller, F.; Chou, L.; Gedge, F.; Tang, W.; Coon, H.; Mao, R. Genotype-phenotype correlation in hereditary hemorrhagic telangiectasia: Mutations and manifestations. *Am. J. Med. Genet.* **2006**, *140*, 463–470. [CrossRef]
5. Shovlin, C.L.; Guttmacher, A.E.; Buscarini, E.; Faughnan, M.E.; Hyland, R.H.; Westermann, C.J.; Kjeldsen, A.D.; Plauchu, H. Diagnostic criteria for hereditary hemorrhagic telangiectasia (Rendu-Osler-Weber syndrome). *Am. J. Med. Genet.* **2000**, *91*, 66–67. [CrossRef]
6. Govani, F.S.; Shovlin, C.L. Hereditary haemorrhagic telangiectasia: A clinical and scientific review. *Eur. J. Hum. Genet.* **2009**, *17*, 860–871. [CrossRef]
7. Shovlin, C.L.; Hughes, J.M.; Tuddenham, E.G.; Temperley, I.; Perembelon, Y.F.; Scott, J.; Seidman, C.E.; Seidman, J.G. A gene for hereditary haemorrhagic telangiectasia maps to chromosome 9q3. *Nat. Genet.* **1994**, *2*, 205–209. [CrossRef]
8. Johnson, D.W.; Berg, J.N.; Baldwin, M.A.; Gallione, C.J.; Marondel, I.; Yoon, S.J.; Stenzel, T.T.; Speer, M.; Pericak-Vance, M.A.; Diamond, A.; et al. Mutations in the activin receptor-like kinase 1 gene in hereditary haemorrhagic telangiectasia type 2. *Nat. Genet.* **1996**, *13*, 189–195. [CrossRef]
9. Gallione, C.J.; Repetto, G.M.; Legius, E.; Rustgi, A.K.; Schelley, S.L.; Tejpar, S.; Mitchell, G.; Drouin, E.; Westermann, C.J.; Marchuk, D.A. A combined syndrome of juvenile polyposis and hereditary haemorrhagic telangiectasia associated with mutations in MADH4 (SMAD4). *Lancet* **2004**, *9412*, 852–859. [CrossRef] [PubMed]
10. Wooderchak-Donahue, W.L.; McDonald, J.; O'Fallon, B.; Upton, P.D.; Li, W.; Roman, B.L.; Young, S.; Plant, P.; Fulop, G.T.; Langa, C.; et al. BMP9 Mutations cause a vascular-anomaly syndrome with phenotypic overlap with hereditary hemorrhagic telangiectasia. *Am. J. Hum. Genet.* **2013**, *93*, 530–537. [CrossRef]
11. McDonald, J.; Wooderchak-Donahue, W.; Van Sant Webb, C.; Whitehead, K.; Stevenson, D.A.; Bayrak-Toydemir, P. Hereditary hemorrhagic telangiectasia: Genetics and molecular diagnostics in a new era. *Front. Genet.* **2015**, *6*, 1–8. [CrossRef]
12. HHT Mutation Database. Available online: https://arup.utah.edu/database/HHT/ (accessed on 5 June 2021).
13. Tørring, P.M.; Brusgaard, K.; Ousager, L.B.; Andersen, P.E.; Kjeldsen, A.D. National mutation study among Danish patients with hereditary haemorrhagic telangiectasia. *Clin. Genet.* **2013**, *86*, 123–133. [CrossRef]
14. Pierucci, P.; Lenato, G.M.; Suppressa, P.; Lastella, P.; Triggiani, V.; Valerio, R.; Comelli, M.; Salvante, D.; Stella, A.; Resta, N.; et al. A long diagnostic delay in patients with hereditary haemorrhagic telangiectasia: A questionnaire-based retrospective study. *Orphanet J. Rare Dis.* **2012**, *7*, 33. [CrossRef]
15. Major, T.; Gindele, R.; Szabó, Z.; Kis, Z.; Bora, L.; Jóni, N.; Bárdossy, P.; Rácz, T.; Bereczky, Z. The stratified population screening of hereditary hemorrhagic telangiectasia. *Pathol. Oncol. Res.* **2020**, *26*, 2783–2788. [CrossRef]
16. Major, T.; Gindele, R.; Szabó, Z.; Alef, T.; Thiele, B.; Bora, L.; Kis, Z.; Bárdossy, P.; Rácz, T.; Havacs, I.; et al. Evidence for the founder effect of a novel ACVRL1 splice-site mutation in Hungarian hereditary hemorrhagic telangiectasia families. *Clin. Genet.* **2016**, *90*, 466–467. [CrossRef]
17. Gindele, R.; Kerényi, A.; Kállai, J.; Pfliegler, G.; Schlammadinger, Á.; Szegedi, I.; Major, T.; Szabó, Z.; Bagoly, Z.; Kiss, C.; et al. Resolving differential diagnostic problems in von willebrand disease, in fibrinogen disorders, in prekallikrein deficiency and in hereditary hemorrhagic telangiectasia by next-generation sequencing. *Life* **2021**, *11*, 202. [CrossRef]
18. Széles, G.; Vokó, Z.; Jenei, T.; Kardos, L.; Pocsai, Z.; Bajtay, A.; Papp, E.; Pásti, G.; Kósa, Z.; Molnár, I.; et al. A preliminary evaluation of a health monitoring programme in Hungary. *Eur. J. Public Health* **2005**, *15*, 26–32. [CrossRef]
19. The Human Gene Mutation Database. Available online: http://www.hgmd.cf.ac.uk/ac/index.php (accessed on 5 June 2021).
20. Møller, P.; Clark, N.; Mæhle, L. A SImplified method for segregation analysis (SISA) to determine penetrance and expression of a genetic variant in a family. *Hum. Mutat.* **2011**, *32*, 568–571. [CrossRef]
21. Franklin by Genoox. Available online: https://franklin.genoox.com/clinical-db/home (accessed on 14 June 2021).
22. Richards, S.; Aziz, N.; Bale, S.; Bick, D.; Das, S.; Gastier-Foster, J.; Grody, W.W.; Hegde, M.; Lyon, E.; Spector, E.; et al. Standards and guidelines for the interpretation of sequence variants: A joint consensus recommendation of the american college of medical genetics and genomics and the association for molecular pathology. *Genet. Med.* **2015**, *17*, 405–423. [CrossRef] [PubMed]
23. Major, T.; Gindele, R.; Szabó, Z.; Jóni, N.; Kis, Z.; Bora, L.; Bárdossy, P.; Rácz, T.; Karosi, T.; Bereczky, Z. A hereditér haemorrhagiás teleangiectasia (Osler–Weber–Rendu-kór) genetikai diagnosztikája. *Orv. Hetil.* **2019**, *160*, 710–719. [CrossRef]
24. Major, T.; Csobay-Novák, C.; Gindele, R.; Szabó, Z.; Bora, L.; Jóni, N.; Rácz, T.; Karosi, T.; Bereczky, Z. Pitfalls of delaying the diagnosis of hereditary hemorrhagic telangiectasia. *J. Int. Med. Res.* **2020**, *48*, 300060519860971. [CrossRef]
25. Lesca, G.; Olivieri, C.; Burnichon, N.; Pagella, F.; Carette, M.F.; Gilbert-Dussardier, B.; Goizet, C.; Roume, J.; Rabilloud, M.; Saurin, J.C.; et al. French-Italian-Rendu-Osler Network. Genotype-phenotype correlations in hereditary hemorrhagic telangiectasia: Data from the French-Italian HHT network. *Genet. Med.* **2007**, *9*, 14–22. [CrossRef] [PubMed]
26. Westermann, C.J.J.; Rosina, A.F.; de Vries, V.; de Coteau, P.A. The prevalence and manifestations of hereditary hemorrhagic telangiectasia in the Afro-Caribbean population of the Netherlands Antilles: A family screening. *Am. J. Med. Genet.* **2003**, *116*, 324–328. [CrossRef] [PubMed]
27. Donaldson, J.W.; McKeever, T.M.; Hall, I.P.; Hubbard, R.B.; Fogarty, A.W. The UK prevalence of hereditary haemorrhagic telangiectasia and its association with sex, socioeconomic status and region of residence: A population-based study. *Thorax* **2014**, *69*, 161–677. [CrossRef] [PubMed]
28. Grosse, S.D.; Boulet, S.L.; Grant, A.M.; Hulihan, M.M.; Faughnan, M.E. The use of US health insurance data for surveillance of rare disorders: Hereditary hemorrhagic telangiectasia. *Genet. Med.* **2014**, *16*, 33–39. [CrossRef]

29. Bossler, A.D.; Richards, J.; George, C.; Godmilow, L.; Ganguly, A. Novel mutations in ENG and ACVRL1 identified in a series of 200 individuals undergoing clinical genetic testing for hereditary hemorrhagic telangiectasia (HHT): Correlation of genotype with phenotype. *Hum. Mutat.* **2006**, *27*, 667–675. [CrossRef]
30. Heimdal, K.; Dalhus, B.; Rødningen, O.K.; Kroken, M.; Eiklid, K.; Dheyauldeen, S.; Røysland, T.; Andersen, R.; Kulseth, M.A. Mutation analysis in Norwegian families with hereditary hemorrhagic telangiectasia: Founder mutations inACVRL1. *Clin. Genet.* **2015**, *89*, 182–186. [CrossRef]
31. Lesca, G.; Plauchu, H.; Coulet, F.; Lefebvre, S.; Plessis, G.; Odent, S.; Rivière, S.; Leheup, B.; Goizet, C.; Carette, M.-F.; et al. Molecular screening ofALK1/ACVRL1andENGgenes in hereditary hemorrhagic telangiectasia in France. *Hum. Mutat.* **2004**, *23*, 289–299. [CrossRef]
32. Lesca, G.; Burnichon, N.; Raux, G.; Tosi, M.; Pinson, S.; Marion, M.J.; Babin, E.; Gilbert-Dussardier, B.; Rivière, S.; Goizet, C.; et al. French rendu-osler network. distribution of ENG and ACVRL1 (ALK1) mutations in French HHT patients. *Hum. Mutat.* **2006**, *27*, 598. [CrossRef]
33. Sabbà, C.; Pasculli, G.; Lenato, G.M.; Suppressa, P.; Lastella, P.; Memeo, M.; Dicuonzo, F.; Guant, G. Hereditary hemorrhagic telangictasia: Clinical features in ENG and ALK1 mutation carriers. *J. Thromb. Haemost.* **2007**, *6*, 1149–1157. [CrossRef]
34. Letteboer, T.G.W.; Zewald, R.A.; Kamping, E.J.; de Haas, G.; Mager, J.J.; Snijder, R.J.; Lindhout, D.; Hennekam, F.A.M.; Westermann, C.J.J.; Ploos van Amstel, J.K. Hereditary hemorrhagic telangiectasia: ENG and ALK-1 mutations in Dutch patients. *Hum. Genet.* **2004**, *116*, 8–16. [CrossRef]
35. Letteboer, T.G.; Mager, J.J.; Snijder, R.J.; Koeleman, B.P.; Lindhout, D.; Ploos van Amstel, J.K.; Westermann, C.J. Genotype-phenotype relationship in hereditary haemorrhagic telangiectasia. *J. Med. Genet.* **2006**, *43*, 371–377. [CrossRef]
36. Olivieri, C.; Pagella, F.; Semino, L.; Lanzarini, L.; Valacca, C.; Pilotto, A.; Corno, S.; Scappaticci, S.; Manfredi, G.; Buscarini, E.; et al. Analysis of ENG and ACVRL1 genes in 137 HHT Italian families identifies 76 different mutations (24 novel). Comparison with other European studies. *J. Hum. Genet.* **2007**, *52*, 820–829. [CrossRef] [PubMed]
37. Sánchez-Martínez, R.; Iriarte, A.; Mora-Luján, J.M.; Patier, J.L.; López-Wolf, D.; Ojeda, A.; Torralba, M.A.; Juyol, M.C.; Gil, R.; Añón, S.; et al. RiHHTa Investigators of the rare diseases working group from the spanish society of internal medicine. Current HHT genetic overview in Spain and its phenotypic correlation: Data from RiHHTa registry. *Orphanet J. Rare Dis.* **2020**, *15*, 138. [CrossRef] [PubMed]
38. McDonald, J.; Bayrak-Toydemir, P.; DeMille, D.; Wooderchak-Donahue, W.; Whitehead, K. Curaçao diagnostic criteria for hereditary hemorrhagic telangiectasia is highly predictive of a pathogenic variant in ENG or ACVRL1 (HHT1 and HHT2). *Genet. Med.* **2020**, *22*, 1201–1205. [CrossRef] [PubMed]
39. Major, T.; Gindele, R.; Balogh, G.; Bárdossy, P.; Bereczky, Z. Founder effects in hereditary hemorrhagic telangiectasia. *J. Clin. Med.* **2021**, *10*, 1682. [CrossRef]
40. Lesca, G.; Genin, E.; Blachier, C.; Olivieri, C.; Coulet, F.; Brunet, G.; Dupuis-Girod, S.; Buscarini, E.; Soubrier, F.; Calender, A.; et al. Hereditary hemorrhagic telangiectasia: Evidence for regional founder effects of ACVRL1 mutations in French and Italian patients. *Eur. J. Hum. Genet.* **2008**, *16*, 742–749. [CrossRef]
41. Plauchu, H.; De Chadarévian, J.-P.; Bideau, A.; Robert, J.-M. Age-related clinical profile of hereditary hemorrhagic telangiectasia in an epidemiologically recruited population. *Am. J. Med. Genet.* **1989**, *32*, 291–297. [CrossRef]
42. Faughnan, M.E.; Palda, V.A.; Garcia-Tsao, G.; Geisthoff, U.W.; McDonald, J.; Proctor, D.D.; Spears, J.; Brown, D.H.; Buscarini, E.; Chesnutt, M.S.; et al. HHT foundation international—Guidelines working group. *International guidelines for the diagnosis and management of hereditary haemorrhagic telangiectasia. J. Med. Genet.* **2011**, *48*, 73–87. [CrossRef]
43. Faughnan, M.E.; Mager, J.J.; Hetts, S.W.; Palda, V.A.; Lang-Robertson, K.; Buscarini, E.; Deslandres, E.; Kasthuri, R.S.; Lausman, A.; Poetker, D.; et al. Second International guidelines for the diagnosis and management of hereditary hemorrhagic telangiectasia. *Ann. Intern. Med.* **2020**, *15*, 989–1001. [CrossRef]
44. Kritharis, A.; Al-Samkari, H.; Kuter, D.J. Hereditary hemorrhagic telangiectasia: Diagnosis and management from the hematologist's perspective. *Haematologica* **2018**, *103*, 1433–1443. [CrossRef]
45. Shovlin, C.L.; Buscarini, E.; Kjeldsen, A.D.; Mager, H.J.; Sabbà, C.; Droege, F.; Geisthoff, U.; Ugolini, S.; Dupuis-Girod, S. European reference network for rare vascular diseases (VASCERN) outcome measures for hereditary haemorrhagic telangiectasia (HHT). *Orphanet J. Rare Dis.* **2018**, *13*, 136. [CrossRef] [PubMed]
46. Ingrosso, M.; Sabbà, C.; Pisani, A.; Principi, M.; Gallitelli, M.; Cirulli, A.; Francavilla, A. Evidence of small-bowel involvement in hereditary hemorrhagic telangiectasia: A capsule-endoscopic study. *Endoscopy* **2004**, *36*, 1074–1079. [CrossRef]
47. Canzonieri, C.; Centenara, L.; Ornati, F.; Pagella, F.; Matti, E.; Alvisi, C.; Danesino, C.; Perego, M.; Olivieri, C. Endoscopic evaluation of gastrointestinal tract in patients with hereditary hemorrhagic telangiectasia and correlation with their genotypes. *Genet. Med.* **2014**, *16*, 3–10. [CrossRef] [PubMed]
48. Pahl, K.S.; Choudhury, A.; Wusik, K.; Hammill, A.; White, A.; Henderson, K.; Pollak, J.; Kasthuri, R.S. Applicability of the curaçao criteria for the diagnosis of hereditary hemorrhagic telangiectasia in the pediatric population. *J. Pediatr.* **2018**, *197*, 207–213. [CrossRef] [PubMed]
49. Kroon, S.; Snijder, R.J.; Faughnan, M.E.; Mager, H.J. Systematic screening in hereditary hemorrhagic telangiectasia: A review. *Curr. Opin. Pulm. Med.* **2018**, *24*, 260–268. [CrossRef] [PubMed]

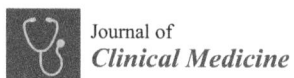

Article

Beneficial Effects of Remote Medical Care for Patients with Hereditary Hemorrhagic Telangiectasia during the COVID-19 Pandemic

Eleonora Gaetani [1,2,*], Fabiana Agostini [1,2], Luigi Di Martino [1,2], Denis Occhipinti [1], Giulio Cesare Passali [1,3], Mariaconsiglia Santantonio [1,3], Giuseppe Marano [1,4,5], Marianna Mazza [1,4], Roberto Pola [1,2] and on behalf of the Multidisciplinary Gemelli Group for HHT [†]

[1] Multidisciplinary Gemelli Group for HHT, Fondazione Policlinico Universitario A. Gemelli IRCCS, Università Cattolica del Sacro Cuore, 00168 Rome, Italy; fabiana.agostini@libero.it (F.A.); luigidimartino7@gmail.com (L.D.M.); denis.occhipinti@gmail.com (D.O.); GiulioCesare.Passali@unicatt.it (G.C.P.); mariaconsiglia.santantonio@policlinicogemelli.it (M.S.); giuseppemaranogm@gmail.com (G.M.); marianna.mazza@policlinicogemelli.it (M.M.); roberto.pola@unicatt.it (R.P.)
[2] Department of Translational Medicine and Surgery, Fondazione Policlinico Universitario A. Gemelli IRCCS, Università Cattolica del Sacro Cuore, 00168 Rome, Italy
[3] Division of Otorhinolaryngology, Fondazione Policlinico Universitario A. Gemelli IRCCS, Università Cattolica del Sacro Cuore, 00168 Rome, Italy
[4] Institute of Psychiatry and Psychology, Fondazione Policlinico Universitario A. Gemelli IRCCS, Università Cattolica del Sacro Cuore, 00168 Rome, Italy
[5] U.P. ASPIC Università Popolare del Counseling, 00145 Rome, Italy
* Correspondence: eleonora.gaetani@unicatt.it; Tel.: +39-06-30157075
[†] Membership of the Multidisciplinary Gemelli Group for HHT is provided in the Acknowledgments.

Abstract: Background: Hereditary hemorrhagic telangiectasia (HHT) needs high-quality care and multidisciplinary management. During the COVID-19 pandemic, most non-urgent clinical activities for HHT outpatients were suspended. We conducted an analytical observational cohort study to evaluate whether medical and psychological support, provided through remote consultation during the COVID-19 pandemic, could reduce the complications of HHT. Methods: A structured regimen of remote consultations, conducted by either video-calls, telephone calls, or e-mails, was provided by a multidisciplinary group of physicians to a set of patients of our HHT center. The outcomes considered were: number of emergency room visits/hospitalizations, need of blood transfusions, need of iron supplementation, worsening of epistaxis, and psychological status. Results: The study included 45 patients who received remote assistance for a total of eight months. During this period, 9 patients required emergency room visits, 6 needed blood transfusions, and 24 needed iron supplementation. This was not different from what was registered among the same 45 patients in the same period of the previous year. Remote care also resulted in better management of epistaxis and improved quality of life, with the mean epistaxis severity score and the Euro-Quality of Life-Visual Analogue Scale that were significantly better at the end than at the beginning of the study. Discussion: Remote medical care might be a valid support for HHT subjects during periods of suspended outpatient surveillance, like the COVID-19 pandemic.

Keywords: hereditary hemorrhagic telangiectasia; COVID-19; telemedicine; remote consultation; epistaxis; quality of life

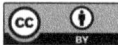

1. Introduction

Hereditary hemorrhagic telangiectasia (HHT) is a dominantly inheritable rare disease, characterized by the presence of multiple arteriovenous malformations (AVMs), leading to a wide variety of clinical manifestations, such us spontaneous and recurrent epistaxis, gastrointestinal bleeding, cerebral abscess or stroke due to paradoxical embolism from pulmonary AVMs, and intracerebral hemorrhage [1,2]. As with many other rare diseases, patients with HHT often experience life-long disability, life-threatening conditions, and a severely impacted quality of life [3,4]. They require many different types of medical services, including emergency rooms visits, urgent laboratory tests, blood transfusions, specific therapies, and psychological support. More generally, they need high-quality care and careful multidisciplinary follow-up and management [5].

Since the beginning of the COVID-19 pandemic, unprecedented public health measures have been undertaken worldwide to reduce the spread of the infection. Many hospitals have reduced or closed healthcare services for outpatients, including screening examinations and follow-up visits for subjects affected by HHT. The burden has been high also at the social and psychological level, especially when associated with the confinement measures imposed by many governments [6,7]. In this scenario, it is mandatory to develop alternative methods to provide assistance to patients, in particular those with peculiar needs [8–12]. In the specific field of rare diseases, the development of telemedicine and remote consultation is fundamental, as many of these patients have been experiencing a feeling of fear and abandon during the COVID-19 pandemic, with many cases of poor compliance to therapy and discontinuation of important treatments [13,14].

In this study, we conducted an analytical observational cohort study to evaluate whether a regimen of medical and psychological support provided to HHT patients through remote consultation during the COVID-19 pandemic has a positive impact on the disease, with reduced need of emergency room visits and hospitalizations, better management of epistaxis, and improvement of quality of life.

2. Materials and Methods

We contacted all patients with a definite diagnosis of HHT by e-mail and/or telephone [15] who had been followed at our HHT center for at least one year and asked them if they were willing to participate to the study. We did not contact patients below the age of 18. The patients who agreed to participate signed an informed consent form. The study started on 1 June 2020 and ended on 31 January 2021. The study was approved by the Ethics Committee of the "Fondazione Policlinico Universitario A. Gemelli IRCCS" (Rome, Italy) (protocol number 0020292/20, ID 3194).

Participating patients received weekly or biweekly clinical evaluations, depending on individual needs, by the means of remote consultations, conducted by either video calls, telephone calls, and/or e-mails. Based on individual needs, clinical evaluations were performed by one or more doctors of the multidisciplinary HHT center, including, among others, specialists in otorhinolaryngology, internal medicine, gastroenterology, neurology, and psychiatry. During remote consultations, doctors evaluated the general conditions of the individual patient, inspected the results of laboratory and radiological exams, provided clinical advices, and, if necessary, prescribed additional tests and medications.

The impact of remote medical assistance was assessed every two weeks until the conclusion of the study by determining the number of emergency room visits and hospitalizations, the need of blood transfusions, and the need of iron supplementation (either intravenous or oral). Results were compared with the data recorded in our electronic database in the same patients in the same period of time of the previous year (1 June 2019–31 January 2020). In order to assess the impact of remote consultation on the management of epistaxis, we recorded the epistaxis severity score (ESS), an internationally recognized score for nosebleed in HHT [16]. The score was measured in each patient at the beginning and at the end of the study. We also assessed the grade of overall health self-perception at the beginning and at the end of the study, using the Euro-Quality of Life-Visual Analogue Scale (EQ-VAS) [17].

SPSS 23.0 was used to perform statistical analysis. Results were expressed as mean ± SD or n (%). Comparisons between groups were made by χ^2 test. p values less than 0.05 were considered statistically significant.

3. Results

A total of 126 patients met the criteria to be included in the study and were asked to participate. Of these, 45 patients (35.7%) accepted. Their demographical and clinical characteristics are presented in Table 1.

Table 1. Characteristics of the study population (n = 45).

Mean age (years ± SD)	56.7 ± 16.1
Gender (male/female ratio)	21/24
ENG pathogenetic mutations (n/screened)	9/37
ACVRL1 pathogenetic mutations (n/screened)	27/37
Epistaxis (n/total)	45/45
Mucocutaneous telangiectases (n/total)	42/45
Family history of HHT (n/total)	45/45
Pulmonary AVMs (n/screened)	17/35
Hepatic AVMs (n/screened)	15/36
Cerebral AVMs (n/screened)	4/34
Previous gastrointestinal bleeding (n/total)	13/45
Anemia at the beginning of the study (n/total)	21/45
Mean Hb levels (g/dL) at the beginning of the study (mean ± SD)	11.7 ± 2.4

There were 21 males and 24 females with a mean age of 56.7 ± 16.1 years. All patients (100.0%) had history of epistaxis. Forty-two patients (93.3%) had mucocutaneous telangiectases. In total, 29 patients (64.4%) had one or more visceral AVMs. There were 17 patients with pulmonary AVMs (on a total of 35 who had been screened for their presence by transthoracic contrast echocardiography or CT scan of the chest), 15 patients with hepatic AVMs (on a total of 36 who had been screened for their presence by either abdominal ultrasound, CT scan, and/or MRI), and 4 patients with cerebral vascular malformations (on a total of 34 who had been screened for their presence by either CT scan and/or MRI of the brain); thirteen patients had history of gastrointestinal bleeding. Genetic tests were available for 37 patients: pathogenic mutations of the ENG gene were present in 9 patients, while pathogenic mutations of the ACVRL1 gene were present in 27 patients. A variant of unknown significance of the ACVRL1 gene was present in one patient. The mean hemoglobin level at the beginning of the study was 11.7 ± 2.4 g/dL.

During the eight-month duration of the study, we recorded the following (Table 2): 9 patients (20.0%) needed emergency room visits and/or hospitalizations; 6 patients (13.3%) needed blood transfusions; and 24 patients (53.3%) needed iron supplementation. There were no significant differences with the same period of the previous year, in which 11 patients (24.4%) needed emergency room visits, 6 patients (13.3%) needed blood transfusions, and 15 patients (33.3%) needed iron supplementation. The only significant difference was the number of patients who received oral iron therapy, which was significantly higher during the period of observation of the study than in the previous year (18/45 vs. 4/45, respectively, $p < 0.02$). Consistently, the number of patients who required intravenous iron infusion during the period of observation of the study (6/45) was lower than the year before (11/45).

Table 2. Outcomes before and during the COVID-19 pandemic.

	June 2019–January 2020	June 2020–January 2021	p
Patients who required emergency room visits or hospitalization, n (%)	11 (24.4)	9 (20.0)	ns
Patients who required blood transfusions, n (%)	6 (13.3)	6 (13.3)	ns
Patients who required iron supplementation, n (%)	15 (33.3)	24 (53.3)	ns
- Oral iron supplementation, n (%)	4 (8.8)	18 (40.0)	<0.02
- Intravenous iron supplementation, n (%)	11 (24.4)	6 (13.3)	ns

Regarding epistaxis (Table 3), we found that the mean ESS was significantly lower at the end than at the beginning of the study (3.0 ± 1.6 vs. 4.4 ± 2.4 respectively, $p < 0.01$). Thirty-two patients (71.1%) reported clinically relevant episodes of epistaxis and required medical advice for the correct management of nosebleed during the study period. The mean ESS was significantly lower at the end than at the beginning of the study also in this subgroup of patients. Indeed, after receiving remote clinical advice about the management of nosebleed through telephone calls and video calls, all these patients reported improvement of symptoms and better epistaxis self-management.

Table 3. Epistaxis severity score (ESS) during the study.

Patients with clinically relevant episodes of epistaxis (ESS ≥ 2) (n/total)	32/45
Mean ESS at beginning vs. at the end of the study:	
- in the study population (mean ± SD)	4.4 ± 2.4 vs. 3.0 ± 1.6 ($p < 0.01$)
- in subjects with clinically relevant episodes of epistaxis (mean ± SD)	5.5 ± 1.9 vs. 3.6 ± 1.4 ($p < 0.01$)

Regarding quality of life, the mean EQ-VAS was 73.1 ± 13.1 at the beginning of the study (Table 4). In the absence of an established pathological threshold for EQ-VAS in HHT patients, we decided to use a value of 70 points to distinguish between subjects with normal and pathological EQ-VAS in our population. This was based on unpublished results from our group that identified 70 points as the median value of EQ-VAS among the HHT patients followed at our multidisciplinary center. Using this threshold, we found 34 patients (75.6%) with EQ-VAS within the normal range and 11 patients (24.4%) with pathological EQ-VAS. Remote psychological support and counselling therapy were offered to the 11 patients with pathological EQ-VAS at the beginning of the study. Five of these patients accepted to adhere while 6 refused. All 5 patients who accepted to receive remote psychological support and counselling therapy reached EQ-VAS values within the normal range by the end of the study. Among the 6 patients who did not accept to receive remote psychological support, only one exhibited normal EQ-VAS value at the end of the study while 3 patients had stable EQ-VAS and 2 had worse EQ-VAS. Regardless of the initial value, 14 patients (31.1%) showed improvement in EQ-VAS at the end of the study compared to the beginning of the study, 25 patients (55.6%) remained stable, and 6 patients (13.3%) reported worsening of EQ-VAS compared to the beginning of the study. Notably, EQ-VAS was higher among the 13 patients who did not have clinically relevant episodes of epistaxis (84.6 ± 8.0 points) compared to the 32 patients with severe epistaxis (70.0 ± 15.7 points). At the end of the study, 18 of the 32 patients with severe epistaxis reported an improvement in EQ-VAS.

Table 4. EQ-VAS values during the study.

Patients with normal EQ-VAS at beginning vs. end of study (n/total)	34/45 vs. 40/45
Patients with pathological EQ-VAS at beginning vs. end of study (n/total)	11/45 vs. 5/45
Mean of EQ-VAS:	
- in the study population (mean ± SD)	73.1 ± 13.1
- in patients with clinically relevant epistaxis (mean ± SD)	70.0 ± 15.7
- in patients without clinically relevant epistaxis (mean ± SD)	84.6 ± 8.0
- EQ-VAS improved at the end of the study (n/total)	14/45
- EQ-VAS stable at the end of the study (n/total)	25/45
- EQ-VAS worsened at the end of the study (n/total)	6/45

4. Discussion

This study is novel and relevant for several reasons. First, it demonstrates that medical care may be provided remotely in an efficacious manner to patients affected by HHT and therefore remote consultations and telemedicine are potential alternatives to classical in-hospital follow-up visits in these patients. Second, it shows that psychological support may be provided remotely with significant beneficial effects. In addition, it provides evidence that correct management of epistaxis can be done at home by patients themselves or their caregivers, without impact on the number of emergency room visits or hospitalization. In addition, anemia may be successfully treated at home, through remote supervision and consultation, with early detection of either hemoglobin decrement and/or iron deficiency and prompt prescription of iron supplementation. Finally, this study demonstrates that personalized regimens of remote consultations have a positive impact on quality of life in HHT patients.

Some aspects of this study deserve additional considerations. One is that remote consultation was associated with a significant increment of the proportion of patients who received a prescription of oral iron supplementation. Indeed, 40% of patients were prescribed oral iron supplementation in 2020, while only 8.8% of them received the same prescription the year before. This was also associated with a concomitant decrease of the proportion of patients who required intravenous iron supplementation (13.3% in 2020 vs. 24.4% in 2019). A possible explanation of this finding is that remote medical consultation, which was provided frequently and periodically in our study, allowed early detection of even small decrements of iron and/or hemoglobin levels and prompt therapeutic intervention. The efficacy of such approach is demonstrated by the fact that the need of blood transfusions was similar between 2019 and 2020, with also no differences in terms of emergency room visits and hospitalizations.

Another aspect that deserves attention is the satisfactory management of epistaxis that it was possible to obtain through remote consultation. Epistaxis is the disorder with the most disrupting effect on the lives of patients with HHT, both at the physical, emotional, social, and professional level [18,19]. In these patients, remote consultation always included a specialist in otorhinolaryngology, who provided practical advice on the best strategies for nasal mucosal care to prevent epistaxis and manage nosebleeds at home, along with the prescription of specific therapies, if needed. It is remarkable that there was a significant improvement of the ESS, not only in the whole study population, but also in those subjects who had clinically relevant episodes of epistaxis at the beginning of the study.

Attention should be paid also to the psychological status of HHT patients, especially in a critical period, such as the COVID-19 pandemic. Social distancing and isolation, combined with fear of contracting COVID-19, could have a significant impact on the psychological status of patients suffering from a rare disease [20]. Moreover, some studies showed that HHT patients could suffer higher levels of psychological distress than the general population, mainly because of chronic anemia and recurrent episodes of nosebleeds [3,4,20,21]. Even in our population, patients without clinically relevant episodes of epistaxis reported significantly higher EQ-VAS values than patients with severe epistaxis. Psychological support through remote consulting and counseling led to the maintenance of the mean values of EQ-VAS of our population within the normal range.

Our study has some limitations. It has a small sample size with a relatively short observation time. However, HHT is a rare disease and the COVID-19 emergency does not allow long observation times. Another limitation is that only about 35% of the patients who were asked to participate accepted to be included in the study. It is possible that these were the most motivated patients and that patients with poor compliance did not agree to participate. This might be a selection bias. Therefore, we are not sure that our results may be applied to the whole HHT population. On the other hand, it is important to point out that many of the patients that were included in the study had complicated HHT phenotypes, including severe epistaxis, chronic anemia, history of gastrointestinal bleeding, and pathological EQ-VAS. Another limitation is that patients who agreed to participate received clinical evaluations which were, in many cases, more frequent than those that they received the year before. Therefore, it cannot be excluded that the clinical improvement that we observed might depend, at least in part, by the frequency of the clinical assistance that was provided to patients and not fully to remote care itself.

In conclusion, this is the first study focused on providing remote medical care to subjects with HHT. Our data show that remote consultation might be a valid support for physicians, caregivers, and patients during periods of suspended surveillance, like the COVID-19 pandemic.

Author Contributions: Conceptualization, E.G. and R.P.; methodology, E.G. and R.P.; software, F.A. and L.D.M.; validation, E.G. and R.P.; formal analysis, F.A. and L.D.M.; investigation, F.A., L.D.M., M.S., G.M., M.M. and D.O.; resources, F.A., L.D.M., M.S., G.M., M.M. and D.O.; data curation, F.A. and L.D.M.; writing—original draft preparation, E.G., F.A., L.D.M. and R.P.; writing—review and editing, E.G. and R.P.; visualization, E.G., G.C.P. and R.P.; supervision, E.G., G.C.P. and R.P.; project administration, E.G., G.C.P. and R.P. All authors have read and agreed to the published version of the manuscript.

Funding: This research did not receive any specific grant from funding agencies in the public, commercial, or not-for-profit sectors.

Institutional Review Board Statement: The study was conducted in accordance with the Declaration of Helsinki, and the protocol was approved by the Ethics Committee of the "Fondazione Policlinico Universitario A. Gemelli IRCCS" (Rome, Italy) (protocol number 0020292/20, ID 3194, approval date 13 May 2020).

Informed Consent Statement: Informed consent was obtained from all subjects involved in the study.

Data Availability Statement: The data presented in this study are available on request from the corresponding author. The data are not publicly available due to ethical and privacy restrictions.

Acknowledgments: Members of the Multidisciplinary Gemelli Group for HHT: Eleonora Gaetani, Giulio Cesare Passali, Maria Elena Riccioni, Annalisa Tortora, Daniela Feliciani, Barbara Funaro, Fabiana Agostini, Leonardo Stella, Luigi Di Martino, Laura Riccardi, Roberto Pola, Angelo Porfidia, Alfredo Puca, Carmelo Sturiale, Aldobrando Broccolini, Marianna Mazza, Giuseppe Marano, Gabriella Locorotondo, Emanuela Lucci Cordisco, Veronica Ojetti, Erica De Candia, Manuel Ferraro, Andrea Contegiacomo, Annemilia Del Cello, Andrea Alexandre, Alessandro Pedicelli, Maria Gabriella Brizi, Silvia D'Ippolito, Fabrizio Minelli, Luigi Corina, Valentina Giorgio, Maria Teresa Lombardi. We are also grateful to Antonio Gasbarrini, Guido Costamagna, Gaetano Paludetti and Giuseppe Zampino for their continuous support to the Multidisciplinary Group.

Conflicts of Interest: The authors declare no conflict of interest.

References

1. Shovlin, C.L.; Buscarini, E.; Kjeldsen, A.D.; Mager, H.J.; Sabba, C.; Droege, F.; Geisthoff, U.; Ugolini, S.; Dupuis-Girod, S. European Reference Network For Rare Vascular Diseases (VASCERN) Outcome Measures For Hereditary Haemorrhagic Telangiectasia (HHT). *Orphanet. J. Rare Dis.* **2018**, *13*, 136. [CrossRef] [PubMed]
2. McDonald, J.; Bayrak-Toydemir, P.; Pyeritz, R.E. Hereditary hemorrhagic telangiectasia: An overview of diagnosis, management, and pathogenesis. *Genet. Med.* **2011**, *13*, 607–616. [CrossRef] [PubMed]
3. Pasculli, G.; Resta, F.; Guastamacchia, E.; Di Gennaro, L.; Suppressa, P. Health-related quality of life in a rare disease: Hereditary hemorrhagic telangiectasia (HHT) or Rendu?Osler?Weber Disease. *Qual. Life Res.* **2004**, *13*, 1715–1723. [CrossRef] [PubMed]
4. Geisthoff, U.W.; Heckmann, K.; D'Amelio, R.; Grünewald, S.; Knöbber, D.; Falkai, P.; Konig, J. Health-Related Quality of Life in Hereditary Hemorrhagic Telangiectasia. *Otolaryngol. Neck Surg.* **2007**, *136*, 726–733. [CrossRef]
5. Faughnan, M.E.; Mager, J.J.; Hetts, S.W.; Palda, V.A.; Lang-Robertson, K.; Buscarini, E.; Deslandres, E.; Kasthuri, R.S.; Lausman, A.; Poetker, D.; et al. Second International Guidelines for the Diagnosis and Management of Hereditary Hemorrhagic Telangiectasia. *Ann. Intern. Med.* **2020**, *173*, 989–1001. [CrossRef]
6. Osofsky, J.D.; Osofsky, H.J.; Mamon, L.Y. Psychological and social impact of COVID-19. *Psychol. Trauma Theory Res. Pr. Policy* **2020**, *12*, 468–469. [CrossRef]
7. Gloster, A.T.; Lamnisos, D.; Lubenko, J.; Presti, G.; Squatrito, V.; Constantinou, M.; Nicolaou, C.; Papacostas, S.; Aydın, G.; Chong, Y.Y.; et al. Impact of COVID-19 pandemic on mental health: An international study. *PLoS ONE* **2020**, *15*, e0244809. [CrossRef] [PubMed]
8. Mann, D.M.; Chen, J.; Chunara, R.; Testa, P.A.; Nov, O. COVID-19 transforms health care through telemedicine: Evidence from the field. *J. Am. Med Inform. Assoc.* **2020**, *27*, 1132–1135. [CrossRef] [PubMed]

9. Smith, A.C.; Thomas, E.; Snoswell, C.L.; Haydon, H.; Mehrotra, A.; Clemensen, J.; Caffery, L.J. Telehealth for global emergencies: Implications for coronavirus disease 2019 (COVID-19). *J. Telemed. Telecare* **2020**, *26*, 309–313. [CrossRef]
10. Boehm, K.; Ziewers, S.; Brandt, M.P.; Sparwasser, P.; Haack, M.; Willems, F.; Thomas, A.; Dotzauer, R.; Höfner, T.; Tsaur, I.; et al. Telemedicine Online Visits in Urology During the COVID-19 Pandemic—Potential, Risk Factors, and Patients' Perspective. *Eur. Urol.* **2020**, *78*, 16–20. [CrossRef]
11. Peretto, G.; De Luca, G.; Campochiaro, C.; Palmisano, A.; Busnardo, E.; Sartorelli, S.; Barzaghi, F.; Cicalese, M.P.; Esposito, A.; Sala, S. Telemedicine in myocarditis: Evolution of a mutidisciplinary "disease unit" at the time of COVID-19 pandemic. *Am. Hear. J.* **2020**, *229*, 121–126. [CrossRef]
12. Sommer, A.C.; Blumenthal, E.Z. Telemedicine in ophthalmology in view of the emerging COVID-19 outbreak. *Graefe's Arch. Clin. Exp. Ophthalmol.* **2020**, *258*, 2341–2352. [CrossRef]
13. Gaetani, E.; Passali, G.C.; Riccioni, M.E.; Tortora, A.; Pola, R.; Costamagna, G.; Gasbarrini, A.; The Multidisciplinary Gemelli Group for HHT. Hereditary haemorrhagic telangiectasia: A disease not to be forgotten during the COVID-19 pandemic. *J. Thromb. Haemost.* **2020**, *18*, 1799–1801. [CrossRef] [PubMed]
14. Riera-Mestre, A.; Iriarte, A.; Moreno, M.; del Castillo, R.; López-Wolf, D. Angiogenesis, hereditary hemorrhagic telangiectasia and COVID-19. *Angiogenesis* **2021**, *24*, 13–15. [CrossRef] [PubMed]
15. Shovlin, C.L.; Guttmacher, A.E.; Buscarini, E.; Faughnan, M.E.; Hyland, R.H.; Westermann, C.J.; Kjeldsen, A.D.; Plauchu, H. Diagnostic criteria for hereditary hemorrhagic telangiectasia (Rendu-Osler-Weber syndrome). *Am. J. Med. Genet.* **2000**, *91*, 66–67. [CrossRef]
16. Hoag, J.B.; Terry, P.; Mitchell, S.; Reh, D.; Merlo, C.A. An epistaxis severity score for hereditary hemorrhagic telangiectasia. *Laryngoscope* **2010**, *120*, 838–843. [CrossRef] [PubMed]
17. Feng, Y.; Parkin, D.; Devlin, N. Assessing the Performance of the EQ-VAS in the NHS PROMs Programme. *SSRN Electron. J.* **2012**, *23*, 977–989. [CrossRef]
18. Merlo, C.A.; Yin, L.; Hoag, J.B.; Mitchell, S.E.; Reh, D.D. The effects of epistaxis on health-related quality of life in patients with hereditary hemorrhagic telangiectasia. *Int. Forum Allergy Rhinol.* **2014**, *4*, 921–925. [CrossRef] [PubMed]
19. Ingrand, I.; Ingrand, P.; Gilbert-Dussardier, B.; Defossez, G.; Jouhet, V.; Migeot, V.; Dufour, X.; Klossek, J.M. Altered quality of life in Rendu-Osler-Weber disease related to recurrent epistaxis. *Rhinol. J.* **2011**, *49*, 155–162. [CrossRef]
20. Marano, G.; Gaetani, E.; Gasbarrini, A.; Janiri, L.; Sani, G.; Mazza, M.; Multidisciplinary Gemelli Group for HHT. Mental health and counseling intervention for hereditary hemorrhagic telangiectasia (HHT) during the COVID-19 pandemic: Perspectives from Italy. *Eur. Rev. Med. Pharmacol. Sci.* **2020**, *24*, 10225–10227. [PubMed]
21. Chaturvedi, S.; Clancy, M.; Schaefer, N.; Oluwole, O.; McCrae, K.R. Depression and post-traumatic stress disorder in individuals with hereditary hemorrhagic telangiectasia: A cross-sectional survey. *Thromb. Res.* **2017**, *153*, 14–18. [CrossRef]

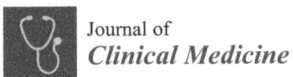

Article

Restless Leg Syndrome Is Underdiagnosed in Hereditary Hemorrhagic Telangiectasia—Results of an Online Survey

Freya Droege [1,*], Andreas Stang [2], Kruthika Thangavelu [3], Carolin Lueb [1], Stephan Lang [1], Michael Xydakis [4] and Urban Geisthoff [3]

1. Department of Otorhinolaryngology, Head and Neck Surgery, University Hospital Essen, University Duisburg-Essen, Hufelandstrasse 55, 45147 Essen, Germany; carolinlueb@googlemail.com (C.L.); stephan.lang@uk-essen.de (S.L.)
2. Institute of Medical Informatics, Biometry and Epidemiology, Essen University Hospital, Hufelandstrasse 55, 45122 Essen, Germany; imibe.dir@uk-essen.de
3. Department of Otorhinolaryngology, Head and Neck Surgery, University Hospital Marburg, Philipps-Universität Marburg, Baldingerstrasse, 35042 Marburg, Germany; kruthika.thangavelu@uk-gm.de (K.T.); urban.geisthoff@med.uni-marburg.de (U.G.)
4. Air Force Research Lab, 2245 Monahan Way, Wright Patterson AFB, Dayton, OH 45433, USA; Michael.Xydakis@us.af.mil
* Correspondence: freya.droege@uk-essen.de; Tel.: +49-201-723-85832; Fax: +49-201-723-1416

Abstract: Background: Recurrent bleeding in patients with hereditary hemorrhagic telangiectasia (HHT) can lead to chronic iron deficiency anemia (CIDA). Existing research points to CIDA as a contributing factor in restless leg syndrome (RLS). The association between HHT-related symptoms and the prevalence of RLS was analyzed. Methods: An online survey was conducted whereby the standardized RLS-Diagnostic Index questionnaire (RLS-DI) was supplemented with 82 additional questions relating to HHT. Results: A total of 474 persons responded to the survey and completed responses for questions pertaining to RLS (mean age: 56 years, 68% females). Per RLS-DI criteria, 48 patients (48/322, 15%; 95% confidence interval (CI): 11–19%) self-identified as having RLS. An analysis of physician-diagnosed RLS and the RLS-DI revealed a relative frequency of RLS in HHT patients of 22% (95% CI: 18–27%). In fact, 8% (25/322; 95% CI: 5–11%) of the HHT patients had RLS which had not been diagnosed before. This equals 35% of the total amount of patients diagnosed with RLS (25/72; 95% CI: 25–46%). HHT patients with a history of gastrointestinal bleeding (prevalence ratio (PR) = 2.70, 95% CI: 1.53–4.77), blood transfusions (PR = 1.90, 95% CI: 1.27–2.86), or iron intake (PR = 2.05, 95% CI: 0.99–4.26) had an increased prevalence of RLS. Conclusions: Our data suggest that RLS is underdiagnosed in HHT. In addition, physicians should assess CIDA parameters for possible iron supplementation.

Keywords: hereditary hemorrhagic telangiectasia; restless leg syndrome; anemia; chronic iron deficiency

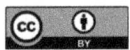

1. Introduction

Hereditary hemorrhagic telangiectasia (HHT) is characterized by systemic visceral arteriovenous malformations and mucocutaneous telangiectasia. Pooled prevalence estimates suggest that HHT occurs in 1 out of 5000–8000 individuals [1]. The etiology is believed to be due to mutations in several genes, (e.g., ENG (HHT Type 1), ACVRL1 (HHT Type 2), SMAD4, and GDF2 (HHT Type 5)) of the transforming growth factor-beta (TGF-β) signaling pathway. These genes play an important role in regulating angiogenesis. Patients often manifest recurrent epistaxis and gastrointestinal bleeding, which may lead to chronic iron deficiency anemia (CIDA) [2,3]. Of note, CIDA is believed to be one of the secondary causes of restless leg syndrome (RLS) [4]. RLS is a movement disorder of unknown etiology that causes an uncontrollable urge to move the lower extremities, particularly during sleep. The underlying pathophysiology of RLS remains unknown, but existing research points to

CIDA as a contributing factor [5,6]. RLS is a commonly overlooked disease with a broad range of severity ranging from mild annoyance to a clinically significant disease severely impairing health and the ability to work [7].

Studies which investigate HHT and its comorbidities are sparse and mostly focused on the effect of larger visceral vascular malformations [8–10]. Chronic iron deficiency and possible secondary diseases related to this are not well studied. To the best of our knowledge this study provides the first analysis of the prevalence of RLS in patients with HHT.

2. Materials and Methods

A survey in German and English was developed and published online (see Supplementary data). Two native English speakers (one otorhinolaryngologist and one patient with HHT), both living in Germany and also fluent in German, translated the questionnaire. Afterwards, 4 authors (U. Geisthoff, F. Droege, K. Thangavelu, and C. Lueb) and another German-speaking HHT patient, crosschecked the translation and optimized it in collaboration with the two native speakers. The survey was disseminated through six different international patient advocacy groups (see acknowledgments). At the end of the survey, some patients provided their email address in case further enquiries should become necessary.

The diagnosis of HHT was established using the modified Curaçao criteria as published by Hosman et al. [11] and Droege et al. [12]. In addition, the general medical history of HHT contained the epistaxis severity score (ESS) for HHT [13]. We also solicited and recorded the need for medical attention, transfusions related to epistaxis, signs of anemia, and hemoglobin levels. RLS was diagnosed using an adapted version of the RLS-Diagnostic Inventory (RLS-DI, see questions 90 to 99 in the Supplementary data), supplemented with 82 additional questions relating to HHT. Patients who stated that they had been diagnosed with RLS by a physician were categorized as "RLS+", and if not, as "RLS−" (see question 85 in the Supplementary data). In addition, according to the RLS-DI, patients were categorized into: "RLS" (score ≥ 11), "no RLS" (score ≤ 1) and "possible RLS" (score between 2 and 10) [14]. Patients who had been diagnosed with RLS by their physician and/or had pathological results in the RLS-DI (categorized as "RLS" or "possible RLS"), were seen as patients with "assumed RLS". The objective of this study was to know what proportion of patients presenting with RLS symptoms (according to the RLS-DI) were actually diagnosed by a physician. Regarding patients with RLS, their medication was documented. Women with an average hemoglobin level below 12.0 g/dL and men with a level below 13.0 g/dL were classified as having anemia [15].

Statistical Methods

Descriptive statistics (number/percentage of patients (N, %) and mean $\pm$ standard deviation (m $\pm$ SD)) were used for the general history of HHT and clinical presentations of HHT-symptoms and RLS diagnosis. The association between ordinal or metric variables were quantified by Pearson's correlation coefficient (r). The association between HHT-related symptoms or medical findings and the prevalence of RLS, was estimated by log-binomial regression models that estimate prevalence ratios (PR) with 95% confidence intervals (CI). Statistical analyses were performed with IBM SPSS Statistics (version 26, Armonk, NY, USA: IBM Corp., released 2019) and SAS® (SAS Institute Inc. 2013. SAS® 9.4 Statements: Reference. Cary, NC, USA: SAS Institute).

3. Results

Study population:

After different international patient advocacy groups informed their members about the online survey, a total of 915 persons responded to it. Evaluation of HHT diagnostic criteria resulted in assignment of 588 with HHT (588/915, 64%, [12]). Not all patients answered all questions which led to smaller subgroups for the following analysis. Of the 588 patients with HHT, 334 (57%, 95% CI: 53–61%) could be contacted via mail and were asked to complete the missing values. Of those patients, 105 provided additional answers (N = 105/334, 31%; 95% CI: 27–37%). Most patients answered the questionnaire for themselves (N = 553/582, 95%; 95% CI: 62–96%), and 29 participants answered for a relative with HHT (N = 29/582, 5%; 95 CI: 4–7%). Not all questionnaires were filled completely, therefore all numbers in the results are given in relation to sufficiently answered questions.

The following data refers to 474 patients with HHT (N = 474/588, 81%; 95% CI: 77–84%) who answered the questions pertaining to RLS. Data from all over the world were collected, and more data came from women with HHT, compared to men (Table 1).

Table 1. Sex and genetic results of patients with HHT.

	Number of Answered Questions (*n* (%))		Number of Patients (*n* (%))
sex	467/474 (99)	males female	148 (32) 319 (68)
genetic testing	468/474 (99)	yes no	260 (56) 208 (44)
genetic mutation	190/474 (40)	HHT Type 1 HHT Type 2 SMAD 4 HHT Type 5	72 (38) 114 (60) 3 (2) 1 (1)

Of the 915 persons who responded to the survey, 588 patients could be diagnosed with hereditary hemorrhagic telangiectasia (HHT) (64%). Of those, 474 patients answered the questions pertaining to RLS (474/588, 81%). There were 467 patients who answered the question about their sex, and 468 patients who stated if they had received a genetic test. In 260 patients a genetic test was performed (N = 260/468, 56%); in 190 patients the result was known. Most patients were females and suffered from HHT Type 2. Data are shown in number of patients (*n*) and percent (%).

Most patients lived in North America or Western Europe (N = 294/339, 87%; 95% CI: 83–90%) Figure 1, and were diagnosed with HHT Type 2 (Table 1). The mean age of patients with HHT was 56 years, with females being younger than males (mean age ± standard deviation (SD): 12 years, range: 20–83 years, N = 149/474, 31%; females: average age = 54 ± 12 years, N = 103/149; males: average age = 60 ± 13 years, N = 46/149).

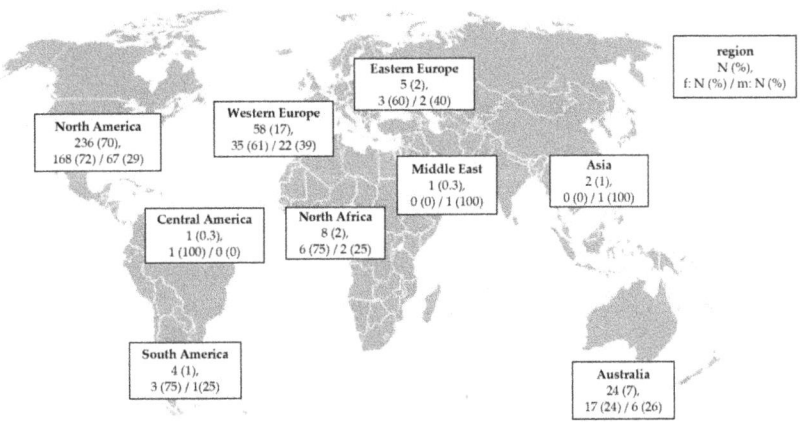

Figure 1. Geographic data of patients with HHT.

In 339 cases who answered the online survey, geographic data of patients with hereditary hemorrhagic telangiectasia (HHT) were documented (N = 339/474, 72%). Most patients came from North America and western Europe (N = 294/339, 87%). Data of sex was obtained in 99% of all patients (N = 335/339). Data are shown in the number of patients (N) and percentage (for all participants, females (f) and males (m)). A free editable world map was used [16].

HHT symptoms:

About 77% of the respondents stated a general progression of HHT (N = 363/473; 95% CI: 73–80%), and 18% (N = 86/473; 95% CI: 15–22%) had a stable disease. Just 5% (N = 24/473; 95% CI: 3–7%) reported a general improvement of the disease. With aging, patients perceived a higher ESS (ESS: r = 0.32; CI: 0.12–0.50). Most patients suffered from recurrent epistaxis (N = 455/474, 96%; 95% CI: 94–97%), and one third from gastrointestinal bleeding (N = 164/453, 36%; 95% CI: 32–41%). The average ESS was 5.8 ($\pm$ 2.2) and the mean hemoglobin level was 10.7 g/dL ($\pm$ 2.7 g/dL). The majority of patients with HHT suffered from anemia (343/425, 81%; 95% CI: 77–84%) and took iron preparations (N = 395/474, 83%; 95% CI: 80–86%; oral alone: N = 217/395, 55%; 95% CI: 50–60%, or parenteral also: 178/395, 45%; 95% CI: 0.40–0.50). There were 134 patients who had received blood transfusions (N = 134/353, 38%; 95% CI: 33–43%; average number of blood transfusions: 17 $\pm$ 48, min: 1, max: 500, median: 5). Hemoglobin levels did not differ between women and men (women (m $\pm$ SD): 10.7 $\pm$ 2.5 g/dL (N = 187/286, 65%); men (m $\pm$ SD): 11.0 $\pm$ 2.7 (N = 99/286, 35%).

Sleep related disorders in patients with HHT:

In 474 cases the RLS-DI question and/or question 85 about RLS-diagnosis by their physician were completed (Figure 2).

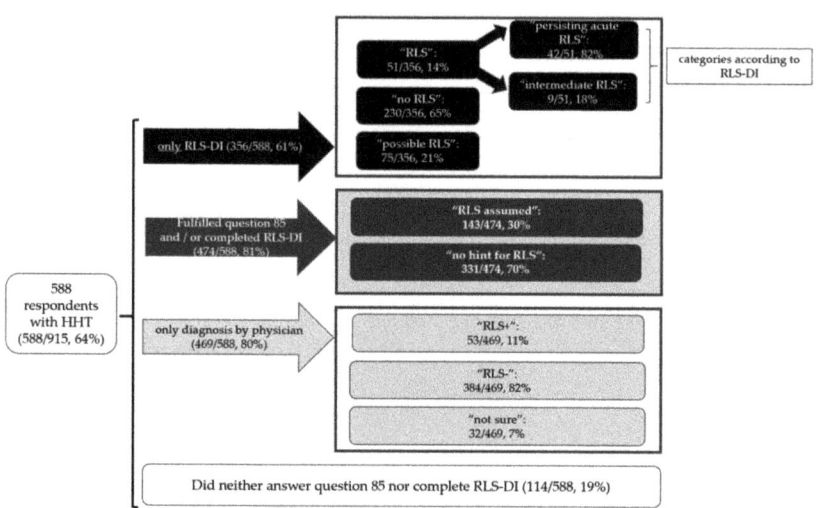

Figure 2. Diagnostic assignment of RLS.

Out of 915 respondents 588 could be diagnosed with hereditary hemorrhagic telangiectasia (HHT; the exact explanation can be found in Figure 2 [12]. There were 469 patients with HHT who stated if their physician had already diagnosed restless leg syndrome (RLS) ("RLS+" = RLS was diagnosed, "RLS-" = no RLS diagnosis; question 85 in Supplementary data), and 356 completed the RLS Diagnostic Inventory (RLS-DI). In 474 cases the RLS-DI and/or the question 85 about RLS-diagnosis by their physician were completed. Here, we assumed RLS in 30% of the patients, as they had been diagnosed by their physician and/or showed a pathological result in the RLS-DI (categorized with "RLS" or "possible RLS"). In only 322 patients with HHT, both the completed RLS-DI AND an answer to question 85 (see Supplementary data), were available (please see Table 2 for further information).

Table 2. RLS-DI questionnaire versus physician diagnosis of RLS.

		Diagnosis by RLS-DI			
		Yes	Possible	No	Sum
RLS diagnosis by physician	yes	23	16	8	47 [a,b]
	no	25 [a,b]	43 [b]	207	275
	sum	48	59	215	322

There were 322 patients with hereditary hemorrhagic telangiectasia (HHT) who answered both, the RLS-DI and the question about the RLS diagnosis by their physician (322/474, 68%). Only the RLS-DI: RLS ("yes"): 48 patients (15%, 95% CI: 12–19%), "possible" RLS: 59 patients (18%, 95% CI: 14–23%), and "no" RLS: 215 patients (67%, 95% CI: 61–72%. Only RLS diagnosis by physician (question 85 in Supplementary data): RLS+ ("yes"): 47 patients (15%, 95% CI: 12–19%), or ("no"): 275 patients (85%, 95% CI: 81–82%). [a] Number of HHT patients with RLS tabulated in the calculation above: (47 + 25)/322 = 72/322 = 22%, 95% CI: 18–27%; of these 72, only 47 (65%, 95% CI: 54–75%) had already been diagnosed by a physician, and 35% (25/72, 95% CI: 25–46%; 8% of 322, 95% CI: 5–11%) had not, respectively. [b] Number of HHT patients with definite and possible RLS counted in the calculations above: (47 + 25 + 43)/322 = 115/332 = 36%, 95% CI: 0.31–0.41; of these 115, only 47 (41%, 95% CI: 32–50%) had already been diagnosed by a physician, and 59% (68/115, 95% CI: 50–68%; 21% of 322, 95% CI: 17–26%) had not, respectively.

Half of the patients with HHT reported that they suffered from a sleep-related disorder in general (N = 206/407, 51%; 95% CI: 0.46–0.55; question 95 in Supplementary data), but just 5% had ever been screened for a sleep-related disorder (N = 19/410; 95% CI: 3–7%; question 98 in Supplementary data). There were 322 patients with HHT who completed the questions about RLS (RLS-DI and question 85 in Supplementary data). Using the RLS-DI, 48 patients (15% of 322 patients; please see also Table 2) were self-identified as having RLS, 33% could be categorized as having (possible) RLS, and 215 (67%) reported no RLS. Yet, when asked whether the presence or absence of RLS was evaluated by a physician, only 15% of the patients responded in the affirmative. Of these patients, 45% received a treatment for their RLS (N = 21/47, 95% CI: 31–59%). An analysis of physician-diagnosed RLS and the RLS-DI, revealed a relative frequency of RLS in HHT patients of 22% to 36% (Table 2, calculations a and b). This value is markedly higher than the historical RLS percentage of 0.8% to 18% in the general population. In fact, 8% (N = 25/322, 95% CI: 0.05–0.11) of the HHT patients had RLS which was not already been diagnosed by a physician. In addition, when "possible RLS" is included, this number increases to 21% (N = 68/322, 95% CI: 17–26%). Therefore, according to our data, between 8% and 21% of the patients with HHT might be underdiagnosed with RLS. These 25 and 68 patients equal 35% and 59%, respectively of the RLS patients of this population (of 72 and 115 patients respectively, when including "possible RLS"; please see also Table 2, calculations a and b). In 8 cases, the patients who had been diagnosed with RLS by their physician before, did not reach a high score in the RLS-DI, possibly due to efficient therapy by medication.

For analyzing the influence of various HHT symptoms and the need of different treatment options, we analyzed patients who we assumed, according to their physician or the RLS-DI, might suffer from RLS ("assumed RLS"; see Materials and Methods section). About one fifth of the HHT patients with anemia also suffered from RLS (N = 63/299, 21%), and patients who had gastrointestinal bleeding (GI) showed an increased prevalence of RLS. In line with this, the patients who needed iron supplementations were more often diagnosed with a neurological disorder. Regarding the diagnosis of RLS, men and women were equally affected and there was no difference in patients' region of origin or genetics (Table 3).

Table 3. Influence of HHT symptoms and patients' characteristics on the prevalence of self-reported RLS.

Symptom	Patients	Assumed RLS *	Percent	PR	95%CI
gastrointestinal bleeding					
no	115	13	11	Ref.	
yes	144	44	31	2.70	1.53–4.77
epistaxis					
no	13	1	8	Ref.	
yes	399	80	20	2.61	0.39–17.31
anemia					
no	71	15	21	Ref.	
yes	299	63	21	1.00	0.60–1.64
blood transfusions					
no	180	31	17	Ref.	
yes	125	41	33	1.90	1.27–2.86
iron intake (oral and/or intravenous)					
no	67	7	10	Ref.	
yes	345	74	21	2.05	0.99–4.26
genetic mutation †					
type 1	59	17	29	1.34	0.77–2.31
type 2	102	22	22	Ref.	
Origin †					
America	213	56	26	Ref.	
Africa	8	4	50	1.90	0.92–3.94
Australia	20	4	20	0.76	0.31–1.88
Europe	52	8	15	0.59	0.30–1.15
sex					
women	274	55	20	Ref.	
men	132	23	17	0.87	0.56–1.35

A total of 474 patients with hereditary hemorrhagic telangiectasia (HHT) answered the RLS−DI and/or if they were diagnosed as having RLS by their physicians. * HHT patients with "assumed RLS", patients who had been diagnosed with RLS, and those as yet undiagnosed with RLS who had pathological results in the RLS−DI (at least "possible RLS" according to the RLS−DI; N = 143/474, 30%; please also see Figure 2). † Because of the small numbers, patients with SMAD4 mutations (N = 1), HHT type 5 (N = 1), and those from Asia (N = 3), were excluded. A log-binominal regression analysis was performed. The number of all patients (Patients) and patients with an assumed diagnosis of RLS (RLS+) are shown. RLS = Restless Legs Syndrome, DI = diagnostic inventory, PR = prevalence ratio, 95% CI = 95% confidence interval, Ref = Reference.

4. Discussion

The historical literature supports an association between HHT and an increased prevalence of neurological disorders. In particular, the reduced pulmonary function as a blood filter in patients with pulmonary arteriovenous malformations, may lead to migraines, cerebral abscesses and strokes [8,17]. Patients with HHT often suffer from recurrent bleeding resulting in a CIDA, which is a recognized cause for restless legs syndrome. However, to our knowledge a potential association between HHT and RLS has not been studied.

In the adult general population, the prevalence of RLS is roughly 0.8–18% [18–20]. Taking into account the patients who had already been diagnosed with RLS and those with a pathologic test result in the RLS−DI, the calculated prevalence of 22–36% for HHT was higher than in the general adult population. According to the literature, about one fourth to one fifth of patients with CIDA exhibit clinically significant RLS [21]. Knowing that CIDA is a common comorbidity in patients with HHT [8] indicates that to diagnose this disease, it might be necessary to ask specific questions about restless legs. Ferri et al. postulated a single question for the rapid screening of RLS (RLS screening: "When you try to relax in the evening or sleep at night, do you ever have unpleasant, restless feelings in your legs that can be relieved by walking or movement?", 100% sensitivity and 96.8% specificity) [22]. In addition, patients with RLS and CIDA often suffer from a sleep-related morbidity [21]. They reported decreased sleep times and had a higher risk for complications like cardiovascular disease [23] and immunological impairment [24]. In our study half of the patients perceived a sleep disorder, but only 5% got further testing. Thus, RLS in HHT is likely underdiagnosed and undertreated. A screening for RLS in HHT patients, especially with CIDA, might be important to prevent comorbidities.

The most common conditions associated with RLS include iron deficiency with low serum ferritin levels, and subsequent low central nervous system intracellular iron [25]. Previous studies indicated that iron deficiency reduces cerebral dopamine receptors and transporters [26]. Alterations in the dopaminergic system may lead to RLS [27]. Anemia is defined by low hemoglobin levels, and patients' iron stores can be measured best by using serum ferritin, indicating the need for iron supplementation [28,29]. In the event of infectious diseases, normal or high ferritin levels do not exclude iron deficiency, as it also acts as an acute phase protein. Here, serum soluble transferrin receptor provides a valuable addition to existing methods, although it is known to be a less specific indicator for iron deficiency than ferritin [30]. Typically, patients with iron deficiency (anemia) aim for normal iron stores and hemoglobin levels. For RLS with CIDA, the iron status is likely to be more important than the anemia [21]. Accordingly, iron treatment reduced RLS symptoms in patients with low serum ferritin levels [26]. Therefore, to treat CIDA in patients with HHT, hemoglobin levels, serum ferritin and maybe soluble transferrin receptors, are important diagnostic markers and should be routinely measured [31]. However, in accordance with another study about CIDA in patients with RLS [21], regarding the RLS diagnosis in patients with HHT there was no relationship between the degree of anemia, iron supplementation, or the need for blood transfusions.

In our study, males and females were equally affected by anemia and RLS. Both, HHT and RLS have been associated with a reduced quality of life and an increased mortality rate [25,32,33]. Treating the underlying condition in CIDA RLS with iron supplementation improves patients' restless legs [34]. Increasing awareness to, or even screening for RLS due to iron deficiency, may therefore improve quality of life and life expectancy of patients with HHT.

Methodological limitations of online-based survey studies warrant consideration. However, multicenter studies with sufficient numbers of patients with HHT are sparse. By questionnaire, patient data obtained from diverse countries can be collected. However, the RLS-DI was not validated for this setting. As we used an English and German version of the survey, most respondents came from North America and Western Europe. Language barriers may be the reason why patients with HHT may not have responded to the survey. Not all patients answered all questions, resulting in a relatively low response rate and smaller subgroups for the analysis. Being an autosomal dominant inherited disease, men and women are equally affected by HHT. In this study, more female patients answered the survey. In general, women are also more prone to RLS than men [35]. In addition, regional differences in the prevalence of RLS exist. Most patients who answered the questionnaire came from Europe and North America where an increased frequency of RLS was reported [36]. We asked if the patients had already been diagnosed with RLS and included the RLS-DI. Other factors also causing RLS (e.g., medication, rheumatoid arthritis, pregnancy, neuropathy and fibromyalgia), iron parameters (e.g., ferritin- or transferrin receptor-level), or a classification of the severity of RLS, were not recorded, and the answers of patients, or diagnoses made by their physicians might have been inaccurate. The RLS-DI is a tool to diagnose actual and persistently present RLS in patients of a sleep laboratory population [14]. The purpose of this study was not to analyze data of sleep laboratories. As we aimed to reach a high number of patients with HHT from all over the world, we relied on patient self-reporting. No direct patient interviews, physical examinations, or evaluation of medical records was performed.

5. Conclusions

In conclusion, we showed for the first time that RLS in patients with HHT is an underdiagnosed and undertreated condition. In particular, patients with recurrent epistaxis and gastrointestinal bleeding had a higher prevalence of RLS. Regular assessment of CIDA parameters and questions about restless legs, as presented in the RLS-DI or mentioned above in patients with HHT, could increase the diagnostic detection probability. Further data are necessary to evaluate if, and what type of screening for RLS in HHT may be justified. Iron supplementation may resolve symptoms of RLS. Thus, paying attention to RLS especially in patients with CIDA may improve patients' quality of life, and even their mortality rate.

Supplementary Materials: The following are available online at https://www.mdpi.com/article/10.3390/jcm10091993/s1, Figure S1: Extracts from the SurveyMonkey questionnaire.

Author Contributions: Conceptualization, F.D. and U.G.; methodology, F.D. and U.G.; software, F.D., C.L. and U.G.; validation, F.D., C.L., K.T. and U.G.; formal analysis, F.D., A.S., C.L., K.T. and U.G.; data curation, F.D. and C.L.; writing—original draft preparation, F.D. and U.G.; writing—review and editing, F.D., A.S., C.L., K.T., S.L., M.X. and U.G.; supervision, U.G. All authors have read and agreed to the published version of the manuscript.

Funding: This research was supported by "Shake the world", Firenze, Italy (UG) and by the University Medicine Essen Clinician Scientist Academy UMEA-Clinician Scientist Program (Deutsche Forschungsgemeinschaft (DFG), project number: 413570972; FD).

Institutional Review Board Statement: All procedures performed in studies involving human participants were in accordance with the 1964 Helsinki declaration (or Declaration of Helsinki) and its later amendments or comparable ethical standards. The study was approved by the Ethics Committee of the University Duisburg-Essen (15-6429-BO; date of approval 19 November 2015). Data were provided voluntarily by the patients.

Informed Consent Statement: Informed consent was obtained from all subjects involved in the study. Data were provided voluntarily by the patients.

Data Availability Statement: Anonymized data will be shared by request from any qualified investigator.

Acknowledgments: The authors are thankful both to the respondents of the survey and the advocacy groups (especially HHTCure, Morbus Osler-Selbsthilfe e.V., HHT Swiss, Osler.DK, Telangiectasia Self Help group, and HHTIreland), for their help with disseminating the questionnaire. In addition, the authors thank Priscilla Meyer and Ralf Schmiedel for assisting in developing the English version of the survey. We acknowledge support by the Open Access Publication Fund of the University of Duisburg-Essen.

Conflicts of Interest: The authors declare no conflict of interest.

References

1. Kjeldsen, A.D.; Vase, P.; Green, A. Hereditary hemorrhagic telangiectasia. A population-based study on prevalence and mortality among Danish HHT patients. *Ugeskr Laeger* **2000**, *162*, 3597–3601. [PubMed]
2. Shovlin, C.L.; Guttmacher, A.E.; Buscarini, E.; Faughnan, M.E.; Hyland, R.H.; Westermann, C.J.; Kjeldsen, A.D.; Plauchu, H. Diagnostic criteria for hereditary hemorrhagic telangiectasia (Rendu-Osler-Weber syndrome). *Am. J. Med. Genet.* **2000**, *91*, 66–67. [CrossRef]
3. McDonald, J.; Wooderchak-Donahue, W.; VanSant Webb, C.; Whitehead, K.; Stevenson, D.A.; Bayrak-Toydemir, P. Hereditary hemorrhagic telangiectasia: Genetics and molecular diagnostics in a new era. *Front. Genet.* **2015**, *6*, 1. [CrossRef] [PubMed]
4. Allen, R.P.; Earley, C.J. The role of iron in restless legs syndrome. *Mov. Disord.* **2007**, *22* (Suppl. 18), S440–S448. [CrossRef] [PubMed]
5. Aspenstroem, G. Pica and Restless Legs in Iron Deficiency. *Sven Lakartidn* **1964**, *61*, 1174–1177.
6. Akyol, A.; Kiyilioglu, N.; Kadikoylu, G.; Bolaman, A.Z.; Ozgel, N. Iron deficiency anemia and restless legs syndrome: Is there an electrophysiological abnormality? *Clin. Neurol. Neurosurg.* **2003**, *106*, 23–27. [CrossRef]
7. Earley, C.J.; Silber, M.H. Restless legs syndrome: Understanding its consequences and the need for better treatment. *Sleep Med.* **2010**, *11*, 807–815. [CrossRef]

8. Droege, F.; Thangavelu, K.; Stuck, B.A.; Stang, A.; Lang, S.; Geisthoff, U. Life expectancy and comorbidities in patients with hereditary hemorrhagic telangiectasia. *Vasc. Med.* **2018**, *23*, 377–383. [CrossRef]
9. Sabba, C.; Pasculli, G.; Suppressa, P.; D'Ovidio, F.; Lenato, G.M.; Resta, F.; Assennato, G.; Guanti, G. Life expectancy in patients with hereditary haemorrhagic telangiectasia. *QJM* **2006**, *99*, 327–334. [CrossRef]
10. Circo, S.; Gossage, J.R. Pulmonary vascular complications of hereditary haemorrhagic telangiectasia. *Curr. Opin. Pulm. Med.* **2014**, *20*, 421–428. [CrossRef]
11. Hosman, A.E.; Shovlin, C.L. Cancer and hereditary haemorrhagic telangiectasia. *J. Cancer Res. Clin. Oncol.* **2017**, *143*, 369–370. [CrossRef]
12. Droege, F.; Lueb, C.; Thangavelu, K.; Stuck, B.A.; Lang, S.; Geisthoff, U. Nasal self-packing for epistaxis in Hereditary Hemorrhagic Telangiectasia increases quality of life. *Rhinology* **2019**, *57*, 231–239. [CrossRef]
13. Hoag, J.B.; Terry, P.; Mitchell, S.; Reh, D.; Merlo, C.A. An epistaxis severity score for hereditary hemorrhagic telangiectasia. *Laryngoscope* **2010**, *120*, 838–843. [CrossRef]
14. Benes, H.; Kohnen, R. Validation of an algorithm for the diagnosis of Restless Legs Syndrome: The Restless Legs Syndrome-Diagnostic Index (RLS-DI). *Sleep Med.* **2009**, *10*, 515–523. [CrossRef]
15. WHO. Haemoglobin concentrations for the diagnosis of anaemia and assessment of severity. In *Vitamin and Mineral Nutrition Information System*; World Health Organization: Geneva, Switzerland, 2011.
16. Softonic. Available online: https://free-editable-worldmap-for-powerpoint.de.softonic.com/ (accessed on 16 September 2020).
17. Post, M.C.; Letteboer, T.G.; Mager, J.J.; Plokker, T.H.; Kelder, J.C.; Westermann, C.J. A pulmonary right-to-left shunt in patients with hereditary hemorrhagic telangiectasia is associated with an increased prevalence of migraine. *Chest* **2005**, *128*, 2485–2489. [CrossRef]
18. Ulfberg, J.; Bjorvatn, B.; Leissner, L.; Gyring, J.; Karlsborg, M.; Regeur, L.; Skeidsvoll, H.; Polo, O.; Partinen, M.; Nordic, R.L.S.S.G. Comorbidity in restless legs syndrome among a sample of Swedish adults. *Sleep Med.* **2007**, *8*, 768–772. [CrossRef]
19. Park, Y.M.; Lee, H.J.; Kang, S.G.; Choi, H.S.; Choi, J.E.; Cho, J.H.; Kim, L. Prevalence of idiopathic and secondary restless legs syndrome in Korean Women. *Gen. Hosp. Psychiatry* **2010**, *32*, 164–168. [CrossRef]
20. Chen, N.H.; Chuang, L.P.; Yang, C.T.; Kushida, C.A.; Hsu, S.C.; Wang, P.C.; Lin, S.W.; Chou, Y.T.; Chen, R.S.; Li, H.Y.; et al. The prevalence of restless legs syndrome in Taiwanese adults. *Psychiatry Clin. Neurosci.* **2010**, *64*, 170–178. [CrossRef]
21. Allen, R.P.; Auerbach, S.; Bahrain, H.; Auerbach, M.; Earley, C.J. The prevalence and impact of restless legs syndrome on patients with iron deficiency anemia. *Am. J. Hematol.* **2013**, *88*, 261–264. [CrossRef]
22. Ferri, R.; Lanuzza, B.; Cosentino, F.I.; Iero, I.; Tripodi, M.; Spada, R.S.; Toscano, G.; Marelli, S.; Arico, D.; Bella, R.; et al. A single question for the rapid screening of restless legs syndrome in the neurological clinical practice. *Eur. J. Neurol.* **2007**, *14*, 1016–1021. [CrossRef]
23. Winkelman, J.W.; Shahar, E.; Sharief, I.; Gottlieb, D.J. Association of restless legs syndrome and cardiovascular disease in the Sleep Heart Health Study. *Neurology* **2008**, *70*, 35–42. [CrossRef] [PubMed]
24. Faraut, B.; Boudjeltia, K.Z.; Vanhamme, L.; Kerkhofs, M. Immune, inflammatory and cardiovascular consequences of sleep restriction and recovery. *Sleep Med. Rev.* **2012**, *16*, 137–149. [CrossRef] [PubMed]
25. Cubo, E.; Gallego-Nieto, C.; Elizari-Roncal, M.; Barroso-Perez, T.; Collazo, C.; Calvo, S.; Delgado-Lopez, P.D. Is Restless Legs Syndrome Associated with an Increased Risk of Mortality? A Meta-Analysis of Cohort Studies. *Tremor Other Hyperkinet Mov.* **2019**, *9*. [CrossRef]
26. Erikson, K.M.; Jones, B.C.; Beard, J.L. Iron deficiency alters dopamine transporter functioning in rat striatum. *J. Nutr.* **2000**, *130*, 2831–2837. [CrossRef] [PubMed]
27. Connor, J.R.; Wang, X.S.; Allen, R.P.; Beard, J.L.; Wiesinger, J.A.; Felt, B.T.; Earley, C.J. Altered dopaminergic profile in the putamen and substantia nigra in restless leg syndrome. *Brain* **2009**, *132*, 2403–2412. [CrossRef] [PubMed]
28. Alvarez-Ossorio, L.; Kirchner, H.; Kluter, H.; Schlenke, P. Low ferritin levels indicate the need for iron supplementation: Strategy to minimize iron-depletion in regular blood donors. *Transfus. Med.* **2000**, *10*, 107–112. [CrossRef] [PubMed]
29. Guyatt, G.H.; Patterson, C.; Ali, M.; Singer, J.; Levine, M.; Turpie, I.; Meyer, R. Diagnosis of iron-deficiency anemia in the elderly. *Am. J. Med.* **1990**, *88*, 205–209. [CrossRef]
30. Means, R.T., Jr.; Allen, J.; Sears, D.A.; Schuster, S.J. Serum soluble transferrin receptor and the prediction of marrow aspirate iron results in a heterogeneous group of patients. *Clin. Lab. Haematol.* **1999**, *21*, 161–167. [CrossRef]
31. Shovlin, C.L.; Buscarini, E.; Kjeldsen, A.D.; Mager, H.J.; Sabba, C.; Droege, F.; Geisthoff, U.; Ugolini, S.; Dupuis-Girod, S. European Reference Network For Rare Vascular Diseases (VASCERN) Outcome Measures For Hereditary Haemorrhagic Telangiectasia (HHT). *Orphanet J. Rare Dis.* **2018**, *13*, 136. [CrossRef]
32. Zarrabeitia, R.; Farinas-Alvarez, C.; Santibanez, M.; Senaris, B.; Fontalba, A.; Botella, L.M.; Parra, J.A. Quality of life in patients with hereditary haemorrhagic telangiectasia (HHT). *Health Qual. Life Outcomes* **2017**, *15*, 19. [CrossRef]
33. Geisthoff, U.W.; Heckmann, K.; D'Amelio, R.; Grunewald, S.; Knobber, D.; Falkai, P.; Konig, J. Health-related quality of life in hereditary hemorrhagic telangiectasia. *Otolaryngol. Head Neck Surg.* **2007**, *136*, 726–733; discussion 734–725. [CrossRef]
34. Wang, J.; O'Reilly, B.; Venkataraman, R.; Mysliwiec, V.; Mysliwiec, A. Efficacy of oral iron in patients with restless legs syndrome and a low-normal ferritin: A randomized, double-blind, placebo-controlled study. *Sleep Med.* **2009**, *10*, 973–975. [CrossRef]
35. Seeman, M.V. Why Are Women Prone to Restless Legs Syndrome? *Int. J. Environ. Res. Public Health* **2020**, *17*, 368. [CrossRef]
36. Koo, B.B. Restless legs syndrome: Relationship between prevalence and latitude. *Sleep Breath* **2012**, *16*, 1237–1245. [CrossRef]

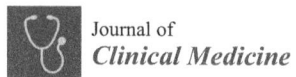

Article

SARS-CoV-2 Infection in Hereditary Hemorrhagic Telangiectasia Patients Suggests Less Clinical Impact Than in the General Population

Sol Marcos [1], Virginia Albiñana [2,3], Lucia Recio-Poveda [2,3], Belisa Tarazona [4], María Patrocinio Verde-González [5,6], Luisa Ojeda-Fernández [2,3] and Luisa-María Botella [2,3,6,*]

1. Otorrinolaringology Department, Hospital Universitario Fundación Alcorcón, 28922 Madrid, Spain; solmarsal70@gmail.com
2. Molecular Biomedicine Department, Centro de Investigaciones Biológicas Margarita Salas, CSIC, 28040 Madrid, Spain; vir_albi_di@yahoo.es (V.A.); luciarecio@hotmail.com (L.R.-P.); mluisa.ojeda@gmail.com (L.O.-F.)
3. CIBER Rare Diseases, U-707, Consortium CIBERER from Carlos III Institute, 28029 Madrid, Spain
4. Preventive Medicine and Public Health Department, Hospital Universitario Fundación Jiménez Díaz, 28040 Madrid, Spain; belimed22@hotmail.com
5. Health Centre Barrio del Pilar, SERMAS, 28029 Madrid, Spain; pverdegonzalez@hotmail.com
6. HHT Spanish Patients Asociation, 28040 Madrid, Spain
* Correspondence: cibluisa@cib.csic.es

Citation: Marcos, S.; Albiñana, V.; Recio-Poveda, L.; Tarazona, B.; Verde-González, M.P.; Ojeda-Fernández, L.; Botella, L.-M. SARS-CoV-2 Infection in Hereditary Hemorrhagic Telangiectasia Patients Suggests Less Clinical Impact Than in the General Population. J. Clin. Med. 2021, 10, 1884. https://doi.org/10.3390/jcm10091884

Academic Editors: Angel M. Cuesta and Süleyman Ergün

Received: 4 April 2021
Accepted: 23 April 2021
Published: 27 April 2021

Publisher's Note: MDPI stays neutral with regard to jurisdictional claims in published maps and institutional affiliations.

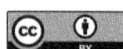

Copyright: © 2021 by the authors. Licensee MDPI, Basel, Switzerland. This article is an open access article distributed under the terms and conditions of the Creative Commons Attribution (CC BY) license (https://creativecommons.org/licenses/by/4.0/).

Abstract: At the moment of writing this communication, the health crisis derived from the COVID-19 pandemic has affected more than 120 million cases, with 40 million corresponding to Europe. In total, the number of deaths is almost 3 million, but continuously rising. Although COVID-19 is primarily a respiratory disease, SARS-CoV-2 infects also endothelial cells in the pulmonary capillaries. This affects the integrity of the endothelium and increases vascular permeability. In addition, there are serious indirect consequences, like disruption of endothelial cells' junctions leading to micro-bleeds and uncontrolled blood clotting. The impact of COVID-19 in people with rare chronic cardiovascular diseases is unknown so far, and interesting to assess, because the virus may cause additional complications in these patients. The aim of the present work was to study the COVID-19 infection among the patients with Hereditary Hemorrhagic Telangiectasia (HHT). A retrospective study was carried out in a 138 HHT patients' sample attending an Ear Nose and Throat (ENT) reference consult. The evaluation of the COVID-19 infection in them reveals milder symptoms; among the 25 HHT patients who were infected, only 3 cases were hospitalized, and none of them required ICU or ventilation assistance. The results are discussed in the light of macrophage immune response.

Keywords: SARS-CoV-2; COVID-19; hereditary hemorrhagic telangiectasia (HHT); pandemic; ACE2 receptor; inflammation; cytokine storm

1. Introduction

At the time of writing this communication, the health crisis derived from the SARS-CoV-2 (COVID-19) pandemic has affected more than 120 million confirmed cases, among these, 40 million corresponding to Europe. In total, almost 3 million deaths have been registered, leading to a sanitary and economic crisis worldwide.

The figures for Spain are 3,136,321 infected and 73,000 deaths, in a total population of 47,351,567. The incidence of infection is then 6.78% of the whole population [1].

The gateway for the infection is the pharyngeal and nasal mucosa, where the virus enters through aerosol transmission or direct contact. The virus penetrates the mucosal epithelium and the endothelium through the ACE2 receptor (angiotensin convertase 2) [2].

This receptor is expressed in different cell types, notably epithelial, fibroblasts, macrophages and vascular endothelial cells.

COVID-19 is also the cause of an endothelial disease, which in the course of its progression would follow the spread in the lower respiratory tract. SARS-CoV-2 binds to the ACE2 receptor and infects endothelial cells in the pulmonary capillaries. This affects the integrity of the endothelium and increases vascular permeability. This vascular damage promotes the development of pulmonary edema and respiratory failure. Next, leukocytes (especially neutrophils) are directed towards the "activated" pulmonary endothelium. Signaling molecules, inflammatory cytokines (generated by the endothelium and the immune system cells) would increase the damage to lung tissue cells by triggering apoptotic processes [3].

In addition to direct damage to the endothelium, there are serious indirect consequences. Disruption of the junctions between endothelial cells can trigger micro-bleeds and uncontrolled blood clotting. On the other hand, blockage of small capillaries by inflammatory cells, coupled with possible thrombosis in larger vessels, can cause ischemia (decreased blood supply) in lung tissue, and even give rise to an uncontrolled inflammatory hyperactivation reaction, the "cytokine storm" [4]. Although inflammation and coagulation are essential defense mechanisms in the body, too much of them can cause irreversible and lethal damage to the patient.

The incidence of COVID-19 in cardiovascular rare diseases is unknown so far, and interesting to assess, because the virus affects the upper and lower airways but also the endothelium, leading to cardiovascular complications. The present communication deals with the incidence of COVID-19 among the patients affected by a rare vascular disease, Hereditary Hemorrhagic Telangiectasia (HHT), in a cohort of patients attending a specialized Ear Nose and Throat (ENT) consult.

Hereditary Hemorrhagic Telangiectasia (HHT) or Rendu-Osler-Weber syndrome is a genetic dominant autosomal multisystemic vascular rare disease, whose penetrance increases with age. The Curaçao criteria represent the clinical diagnosis of HHT, including its main symptoms: spontaneous and recurrent epistaxis (nose bleeds), mucocutaneous telangiectases, visceral localization (gastrointestinal telangiectases and/or arteriovenous malformations (AVMs), mainly in lung, brain or liver, and a first-degree family member with a definite diagnosis of HHT [5–7]. The prevalence of HHT varies between 1:5000 and 1:8000 on average, although because of the "founder effect" and "insulation effect", the prevalence is higher in some regions such as the Jura region in France, Funen Island in Denmark and the Caribbean Dutch Antilles [7–9]. Heterozygous mutations in either *ENDOGLIN (ENG)* or *ACVRL1/ALK1* genes trigger the pathogenesis of HHT in over 90% of HHT patients [10,11]. Mutations in *ENDOGLIN* lead to HHT1 whereas in *ACVRL1* cause HHT2. With 93% of patients suffering light to moderate bleedings, epistaxis presents is the most frequent clinical manifestation of HHT [12–14]. It affects over 90% of patients before the age of 21, normally interfering with their quality of life and leading to chronic anemia. Epistaxis is due to the telangiectases of the nasal mucosa, focally dilated venules, often connected directly with dilated arterioles [15].

The aim of the present work was to study the COVID-19 infection in a cohort of 138 HHT patients attending an Ear Nose and Throat (ENT) reference doctor for HHT. HHT is a rare disease, but the ENT is the specialist visited most frequently for the epistaxis. We wanted to describe the clinical and demographic characteristics of the HHT patients affected by COVID-19, and whether there was any relation between HHT type 1 or 2 and SARS-CoV-2 infection.

2. Materials and Methods

2.1. Population under Study

The present analysis represents a retrospective observational study of a 138 cohort of HHT patients who belong to the ENT reference HHT consult, of the Health Care Provider (HCP), University Hospital, Alcorcon Foundation, (HUFA) of Madrid, Spain.

The collection of the data corresponds to the 11 first months of the pandemic (from March 2020 to February 2021). The incidence of COVID-19, among the HHT group belonging to the ENT consult, was assessed by answering a quick questionnaire, either by e-mail or by phone calls. The idea of performing such a survey came after a Webinar on HHT and COVID-19, organized by the HHT Spain patient association. Patients were previously informed about the study and signed an informed consent form. Variables collected included: sex, age, type of HHT genetic diagnosis (type 1 or 2), HHT-ESS (HHT-Epistaxis Severity Score) presence of arteriovenous malformations (AVMs), COVID-19 diagnosis, and symptoms of the SARS-CoV-2 infection, including hospitalization. Not all the patients received PCR testing, only those with symptoms or those being asymptomatic but in direct contact with relatives or friends tested positive to SARS-CoV-2. The patients diagnosed as positive of COVID-19 obtained the result by PCR; only in one case was diagnosis assessed by a serological test.

2.2. ELISA (Enzyme-Linked Immune Adsorbent Assay) for Detection of Inflammatory Cytokines in Macrophages of HHT Patients

The data provided for ELISA and qPCR analysis were not obtained from macrophages of patients during the COVID-19 pandemic. These data belong to RNA and culture supernatants collected before the pandemic, and belonging to an HHT sample collection of the group of research. Samples of 10 mL from peripheral blood were extracted in EDTA anticoagulant tubes after informed consent of the patients. Proteins studied were: Activin A (DAC00B), CCL20/MIP-3 α (DM3A00), IL-1β (DLB50), IL-6 (D6050), IL-12p40 (DP400), TSP-1 (DTSP10) (R&D Systems).

The detection of proteins in solution (cell culture supernatants) was performed by quantitative ELISA (Enzyme-linked immunoadsorbent assay). Commercial Quantikine® Colorimetric Sandwich ELISA kits from R&D Systems (Minneapolis, MN, USA), whose reference is listed in the following table, were used. Cytokines' production in the supernatant of cell cultures' macrophages from HHT patients and healthy donors were analyzed after treatment with 10 ng/mL of LPS. Levels of IL-1β, IL-12p40, IL6, CCL20, TSP-1 and Activin A released into the supernatant after 48 h of culture were measured. Optical density was determined using a GloMax® Multi Detection System microplate reader (Promega, Madison, WI, USA) with a 450 nm filter. The background correction wavelength was set at 540 nm, following the manufacturer's instructions.

2.3. Analysis of ACE2 Expression by RT-qPCR

Cellular RNA was extracted from macrophages treated with LPS of 10 ng/mL in culture using the commercial kit NucleoSpin® RNA II (Macherey-Nagel, Düren, Alemania). A total of 600 ng of total RNA was subjected to reverse transcription using the First Strand cDNA Synthesis (Roche, Mannheim, Germany), and random primers. Quantitative RT-PCR was performed from 2 microliters of cDNA, and as housekeeping gene, Actin was used. The iQTM SYBR® Green Supermix (Bio-Rad, Herts, UK) was used for the quantitative PCR. ACE2 gene was amplified with the following primers designed according to the software program of the Universal Probe Library: β-actin Fwd: 5′-AGCCTCGCCTTTGCCGA-3′; β-actin Rev: 5′-CTGGTGCCTGGGGCG-3′, ACE-2 Fwd: 5′-TCCATTGGTCTTCTGTCACCCG-3′; ACE-2 Rev: 5′-AGACCATCCACCTCCACTTCTC-3′.

2.4. Statistical Analysis

Qualitative variables are presented with their frequency distributions. For quantitative variables, the mean and standard deviation were calculated. Quantitative variables were compared by the Student's t-test; being statistically significant, those differences where $p < 0.05$. In the Figures 1 and 2, they are represented as follows: * $p < 0.05$ ** $p < 0.01$ *** $p < 0.001$. Statistical analyses were carried out with the software SPSS Windows version 11.0.0 (SPSS Inc., Chicago, IL, USA).

3. Results

3.1. SARS-CoV-2 Infection Data among a Cohort of 138 HHT Patients

The HHT patients attending the ENT consult of HUFA come from all over Spain, and they are representative of the clinical spectrum of HHT patients in Spain, concerning type of HHT, the degree of visceral involvement (AVMs) and a broad range of HHT-ESS, from severe to mild [16]. Data from the whole group of 138 patients attending the ENT reference consult are not, in general, different from the 25 HHT patients who tested positive for COVID-19, concerning the degree of HHT symptoms. As seen in Table 1, data from each single positive COVID-19 patient are shown. The range of all the considered parameters: age, sex ratio, the HHT1 vs. 2 ratio, and the presence of AVMs in these COVID-19-positive patients are not different from the whole group of patients. In particular, in Table 1, we may see 36% patients with pulmonary AVMs (PAVMs), 76% with hepatic AVMs (HAVMs), 4% cerebral AVMs. PAVMs were predominant in HHT1 (75%) vs. HHT2 (17.6%) (Table 1). These frequencies, the same as sex ratio, and prevalence of HHT2 vs. HHT1are within the range of those reported for Spain (RiHHTa Registry) including 211 patients with a mean age of 42 [17].

These patients are currently followed at the ENT consult, by sclerotherapy and propranolol cream on demand [16]. Some of them require additional treatments as mentioned in Table 1. The demographic results of the COVID-19-positive HHT population are shown in Table 2.

Table 1. HHT characteristics and COVID-19 symptoms in the affected group. Results related to HHT symptoms in the positive COVID-19 cases, and the COVID-19 infection derived symptoms.

Patient	Gender	Gene	Type	AVMS	HHT-ESS	Age	Symptoms	Hospital
#1	♀	ENG	HHT1	HAVM	0.91	37	asymptomatic	-
#2	♂	ENG	HHT1	PAVM, HAVM	1.41 $^\alpha$	74	asymptomatic	-
#3	♀	ALK1	HHT2	HAVM	1.01	57	headache, diarrhea	-
#4	♂	ALK1	HHT2	HAVM	1.91	64	headache, diarrhea, myalgias	-
#5	♂	ENG	HHT1	PAVM, HAVM	0.51	70	cough, shortness of breath	-
#6	♂	ALK1	HHT2	HAVM	7.46 $^\varepsilon$	63	suspected diarrhea, serologic detection months later	-
#7	♀	ALK1	HHT2	HAVM	3.51	63	myalgias, headache, nosebleed, diarrhea	-
#8	♂	ALK1	HHT2	-	0.0	29	asymptomatic	-
#9	♀	ENG	HHT1	PAVM, CAVM, HAVM	1.41	32	asymptomatic	-

Table 1. Cont.

Patient	Gender	Gene	Type	AVMS	HHT-ESS	Age	Symptoms	Hospital
#10	♀	ALK1	HHT2	PAVM, HAVM	2.43	47	pneumonia, cough, dyspnea	YES
#11	♀	ALK1	HHT2	HAVM	1.41	56	asymptomatic	-
#12	♀	ENG	HHT1	PAVM, HAVM	1.41	62	asymptomatic	-
#13	♀	ALK1	HHT2	HAVM	3.33	70	asymptomatic	-
#14	♀	ALK1	HHT2	HAVM	5.18 $^\gamma$	87	pneumonia, anemia	YES
#15	♂	ALK1	HHT2	HAVM	0.0	55	headache, diarrhea	-
#16	♀	ALK1	HHT2	-	0.0	25	anosmia, headache	-
#17	♀	ALK1	HHT2	PAVM, HAVM	3.33	50	anosmia, headache, diarrhea	-
#18	♀	ENG	HHT1	PAVM, HAVM	3.33	52	pneumonia, no dyspnea	YES
#19	♀	ENG	HHT1	PAVM, SpAVM	0.0	16	asymptomatic	-
#20	♀	ENG	HHT1	HAVM	2.43 $^\Delta$	49	anosmia, ageusia, moderate fever and slight muscular pain, diarrhea	-
#21	♂	ALK1	HHT2	-	0.0	41	anosmia, ageusia, moderate fever and slight muscular pain	-
#22	♂	ALK1	HHT2	-	0.0	18	infected twice, rhinitis	-
#23	♀	ALK1	HHT2	HAVM	0.51	50	tonsil and ear infections, cough, fever, pain in the chest, and low oxygen saturation (91%)	-
#24	♀	ALK1	HHT2	-	0.0	16	fever, vomit, tiredness and breathless	-
#25	♂	ALK1	HHT2	HAVM	0.0	63	anosmia, headache	-

$^\alpha$ #2 at the beginning, need transfusions; in the last year, no need of transfusions. $^\varepsilon$ #6 dependent on transfusions before Young's procedure. Reopening of Young's in the last year, bleeding but no need of transfusions yet. $^\gamma$ #14 chronic anemia, needed transfusion upon hospitalization. $^\Delta$ #20, treated with low dose of tacrolimus and sclerotherapy. Before, she was transfusion-dependent.

Table 2. Characteristics of patients with HHT and COVID-19. Results in percentages of the different demographic characteristics of the affected population. * Figures represent mean (±SD).

	HHT1 n (%)	HHT2 n (%)
	Sex	
Male	2 (25)	7 (41.1)
Female	6 (75)	10 (58.8)
Age	49 (±19.9) *	49.3 (±19.6) *
	Symptoms	
No	5 (62.5)	3 (18.8)
Yes	3 (37.5)	14 (81.2)
	Hospitalization	
No	7 (87.5)	15 (87.5)
Yes	1 (12.5)	2 (12.5)

The frequency of positive COVID-19 HHT patients was 18.11%, with an average of age of 49 ± 18.9 years. Among the affected patients, 64% were women, and 36% men. Concerning the clinical symptoms of COVID-19-positive patients, 68% had symptoms, mostly mild/moderate, and 32% remained asymptomatic. Only 3 patients (12%) were admitted in hospital, due to pneumonia symptoms, but without needing ventilation or the intensive care unit (ICU). It is noteworthy mentioning that one of the patients was in hospital due to a serious anemia, with need of transfusions, but as a consequence of her chronic anemia due to HHT, than by COVID-19 infection. Considering in detail the symptoms shown by the 18 patients, cough was the most frequent (35.3%), followed by dyspnea (29.4%) and diarrhea (29.4%), myalgia (23.5%), headache (17.6%), fever (11.8%) and anosmia/disgeusia (11.8%). Among the COVID-19-positive patients, 68% were HHT2 and 32% were HHT1. This distribution is similar to the distribution of HHT1 versus HHT2 patients in the ENT consult, and also in agreement with the Spanish ratio with the HHT2 predominance over HHT1 [18], characteristic of Mediterranean countries. Thus, the type of HHT does not seem to affect the frequency, nor the degree of severity of the infection. All data are summarized in Table 1. In general, it does not seem to be an evident relation of HHT symptoms and COVID-19 symptoms, however, in the case of the patient with chronic anemia, COVID/SARS-CoV2 infection increased bleeding, and she required blood transfusions and hospitalization.

COVID-19 incidence in Spanish population is currently at 6.78% [19] while in our descriptive study, the COVID-19 frequency in HHT patients was 18.11%. However, these percentages are not directly comparable. The ratio should be obtained within the total HHT Spanish population, and the results are from a sample of 138 HHT. The incidence appears higher than the whole population because the rate of testing is also higher >10%. This is because the chronic condition of HHT leads to a closer clinical follow-up than in the general population. It is noteworthy mentioning that 8 out of 25 patients were asymptomatic (32%), similar to the general population asymptomatic percentage, range (21.9–35.8%). It is notorious that the percentage of hospitalizations in our study was very low, only 3 cases (12%), while in the general population, it was 40% [19]. Moreover, most importantly, only 3 cases of pneumonia were present, but without need of ventilation in the ICU. In our sample population, the most frequent symptoms were respiratory (cough and dyspnea) and digestive (diarrhea), similar to the general population. It is also noteworthy mentioning the case of one patient infected twice but asymptomatic. Regarding the treatments, people at home were only treated with paracetamol 1 g every 8 h. In the cases of pneumonia, antibiotic was added to prevent/treat concomitant bacterial infection. Altogether, the conclusion to draw is that while we cannot say that the rate of infection is different to the general population, the severity of COVID-19 seems clearly weaker.

3.2. ACE2 Expression in HHT and Control Macrophages

The incidence among HHT does not seem to be less than in the general population, since 25 cases were recorded in a cohort of 138 patients. Nonetheless, the expression of ACE2 receptors was studied, in HHT and control macrophages. To this purpose, real-time RT-qPCRs for ACE2 were performed in macrophages of 3 HHT1, 4 HHT2, and 4 control independent sample donors. At similar cycle for the Actin as housekeeping gene, no significant differences were found among them (Figure 1). In this figure, the higher Cycle threshold (Ct), the less is the expression of ACE2. The Ct of ACE2 ranges from 32.5 to 36 in all samples. The Ct in the case of HHT1 were more homogenous around 35.6, showing less expression than in HHT2 ($p < 0.02$), but similar to control donors. Differences among controls and HHT were not statistically significant.

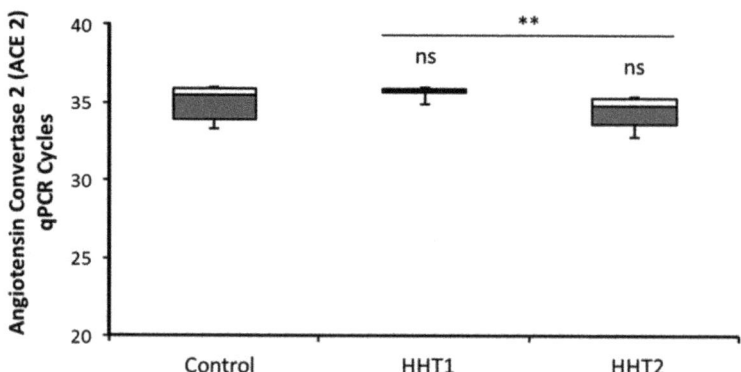

Figure 1. RT-qPCR of Angiotensin Convertase Enzyme type 2 in macrophages of HHT1, HHT2 and Control donors. Mononuclear cells from healthy and HHT donors were cultivated in DMEM with 10% FCS, and treated by LPS 10 ng/mL for 48 h. Cells were lysed, and RNA was extracted as described in Materials and Methods. RT-qPCR was performed for ACE2 receptor in 4 HHT2, 3 HHT1 and 4 control donor samples. Figure represents the number of cycles corresponding to the Ct of the amplification curve at similar Actin RNA amount taken as housekeeping gene. Ns—not significant; ** $p < 0.01$.

3.3. Inflammatory Cytokines in HHT and Control Macrophages

Inflammatory response of macrophages to LPS, in HHT and control patients was analyzed as key factor involved in the so-called cytokine storm triggered by COVID-19 infection in many cases [4]. One way to assess in vitro the inflammatory response in HHT patients versus non-HHT is measuring the production of pro-inflammatory cytokines/chemokines pertinent to the cytokines observed as elevated in COVID-19 patients. For this purpose, mononuclear cells from peripheral blood were cultured from 10 HHT patients (including 5 HHT1 and 5 HHT2), and 10 control donors. The cells were cultured for 48 h in medium supplemented with LPS to induce the inflammatory response. The levels of IL-1β, IL-6, IL-12p40, and CCL20, secreted by the cells were measured by ELISA. In addition, the levels of TSP-1 (Thrombospondin), and the production of Activin A, which is of added interest, as involved in the pro-inflammatory response, were measured [20]. There were no significant differences between HHT1 and HHT2, therefore, the HHT population data were pooled versus control donors. The levels of the selected cytokines (IL-6, IL-1β, IL12p40), CCL20 and TSP-1 were decreased in HHT patients compared to the healthy donors (Figure 2). Similarly, a deficiency in Activin A production after LPS stimulation was observed in cells from HHT patients. In all cases, differences are statistically significant, with decreases of more than 50% for IL-6, IL-1β, IL12p40 and around 50% for CCL20, TSP-1 and Activin A. This significant decrease in inflammatory cytokines detected in the HHT population may explain, at least, partially, the low number of hospitalized patients (only 3 among 25), the absence of acute symptoms, and the lack of needs of ICU, and mechanical ventilation.

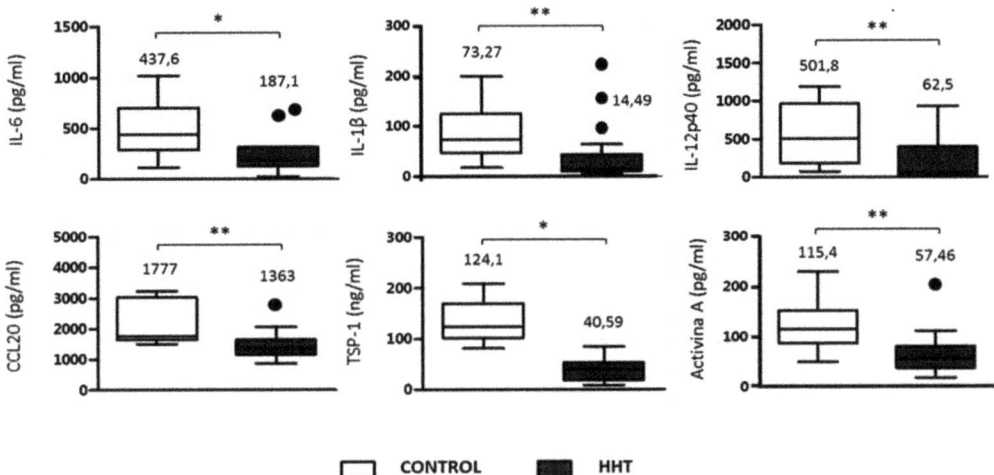

Figure 2. Inflammatory cytokines' analysis in culture media of macrophages, isolated from HHT and control donors. A total of 500,000 mononuclear cells from healthy and HHT donors were cultivated in DMEM with 10% of FCS, and treated by 10 ng/mL of LPS for 48 h. The production of cytokines/chemokines was measured by the corresponding ELISA kits, as described in Materials and Methods. * $p < 0.05$; ** $p < 0.01$.

4. Discussion

There are three essential points to control the pandemic situation caused by SARS-CoV-2: (i) the early diagnosis to prevent the spread of the virus; (ii) the search for effective and safe treatments, essential to reduce the morbidity and mortality of the virus, and (iii) the development of quick vaccination plans to provide the population with immunity against the virus. Ayres (2020) [3] describes 4 phases during infection with COVID-19. Phase 1 presents a moderate symptomatology with fever, discomfort, and dry cough. Phase 2 is characterized by pneumonia with or without hypoxia. As the disease progresses, patients will develop acute respiratory syndrome with multi-organ failure and immune shock (Phase 3). Patients who recover from infection (Phase 4) show a phenotype of resistance, although some of them will never return to their normal pre-infection state (COVID persistence) [21].

The fact of having been diagnosed from HHT does not confer per se an increased risk for SARS-CoV-2 infection. On the other hand, the presented data rather suggest that the HHT patients infected by SARS-CoV-2 do not suffer a more severe infection than the general population, but rather the contrary. The degree of the COVID-19-derived infection symptoms in the HHT sample group studied seemed milder. We will try to discuss the possible factors explaining the COVID-19 less severe symptoms among HHT patients. As a previous reference, Riera et al. [22] reported only one case of a HHT2 COVID-19-positive patient admitted to hospital, in Spain, after the first wave of 2020. The patient was a woman of 74 years, and was hospitalized due to a COVID-19-derived pneumonia. Her clinical course did not involve mechanical ventilation, and she was successfully discharged after two weeks. In this letter [22], the authors refer to this case as the only HHT case admitted in hospital among the RiHHTa (Computerized Spanish Registry of Hereditary Hemorrhagic Telangiectasia). The authors hypothesize that the condition of HHT leads to a damaged endothelium with inflammation and an abnormal angiogenesis which would impair the SARS-CoV-2 infection. This fact would explain the mild clinical symptoms of COVID-19 in HHT patients.

To gain further insight into the COVID-19-HHT relationship, we have explored other factors which may have contributed to the degree of COVID-19 infection in this disease. On one hand, the ACE2 receptor expression and on the other hand, the amount of inflammatory cytokines secreted by HHT macrophages compared with control macrophages. ACE2 that is abundantly expressed in the lungs, the heart, and other tissues is used by SARS-CoV-2 as a functional receptor for their entrance into the cells [23]. The incidence among HHT does not seem to be less than in the general population. Nonetheless, the expression of ACE2 receptors in macrophages was studied, and the results revealed that there are no significant differences between control and HHT macrophages.

Another factor to take into account when examining the severity of the COVID-19 infection is the exacerbation of the inflammatory response triggered by the virus which has been defined as cytokine storm, on the immune system. The inflammatory response of control and HHT macrophages were analyzed, preferentially selecting those inflammatory cytokines reported as involved in the cytokine storm. This acute proinflammatory response damages tissues, including endothelium and contributes to the severity of the disease. The levels of the selected cytokines (IL-6, IL-1β, IL12p40), CCL20 and TSP-1 were decreased in HHT macrophages compared to the healthy donors (Figure 2). Similarly, a deficiency in Activin A production after LPS stimulation was observed in cells from HHT patients. In all cases, differences are statistically significant, with decreases of around or more than 50% in HHT samples. The pathogenesis of the acute pulmonary injury related to COVID-19 is similar to that occurring in other disorders that induce hyperinflammatory state with a release of high amounts of pro-inflammatory cytokines, mainly, IL-1, IL-6 and TNF-α. Thus, drugs that usually serve to treat rheumatic or autoimmune syndromes may play a major role in this setting [24]. In the presence of severe COVID-19 infection, targeted therapies are needed. The use of drugs with therapeutic properties already used for other therapeutic purposes, and which can therefore immediately enter clinical trials because their side effects are known, has been the strategy employed during the pandemic, or what is known as therapeutic drug repositioning [25]. With this goal of repositioning, WHO promoted the SOLIDARITY trial, which has been the largest global (30 countries) randomized drug versus control strategy. The 6-month interim analysis (15 October) indicates that remdesivir, hydroxychloroquine, lopinavir/ritonavir and interferon appear to have little or no effect on mortality or disease course [26]. Notably, Dexamethasone is the only approved drug for the treatment of severe COVID-19 patients who require oxygen therapy (from supplemental oxygen to mechanical ventilation) [27]. Therefore, there is an urgent need to continue the search for new repositioning drugs for immediate use in the absence of targeted treatment. Based on the data of this study, no further analysis regarding special treatment options in HHT could be made.

Nowadays, it is well known that COVID-19 poor prognosis is related to the most common comorbidities as hypertension, obesity, and diabetes [28]. Since in many cases, drugs which decrease cytokines, as corticoids and tocilizumab, had been used to improve the COVID-19 condition; in a way, HHT patients would be naturally producing less cytokines. Thus, without need of these treatments upon SARS-CoV-2 infection, HHT condition would avoid or smooth the acute phase, explaining the milder infections suffered by them.

In this sense, Figure 3 represents a graphical hypothesis of immune response in HHT and control population highlighting the decreased cytokine storm triggered in HHT patients after COVID-19 infection. We believe this may be, among other factors, a crucial point to explain the milder symptoms detected in HHT. In a similar way, we could hypothesize that patients with autoimmune diseases under anti-inflammatory treatment might be, to a certain extent, protected from the severe phases of COVID-19. This hypothesis should be analyzed when data from autoimmune disease cohorts and the COVID-19 infections will be published. On the other hand, in a mouse model KO for endoglin in the myeloid linage, KO mice were protected compared to their wild type and heterozygote littermates, following an in vivo septic shock by LPS. In fact, the survival was higher, and the first deaths were delayed by 36 h compared to their wild type littermates' linage [29].

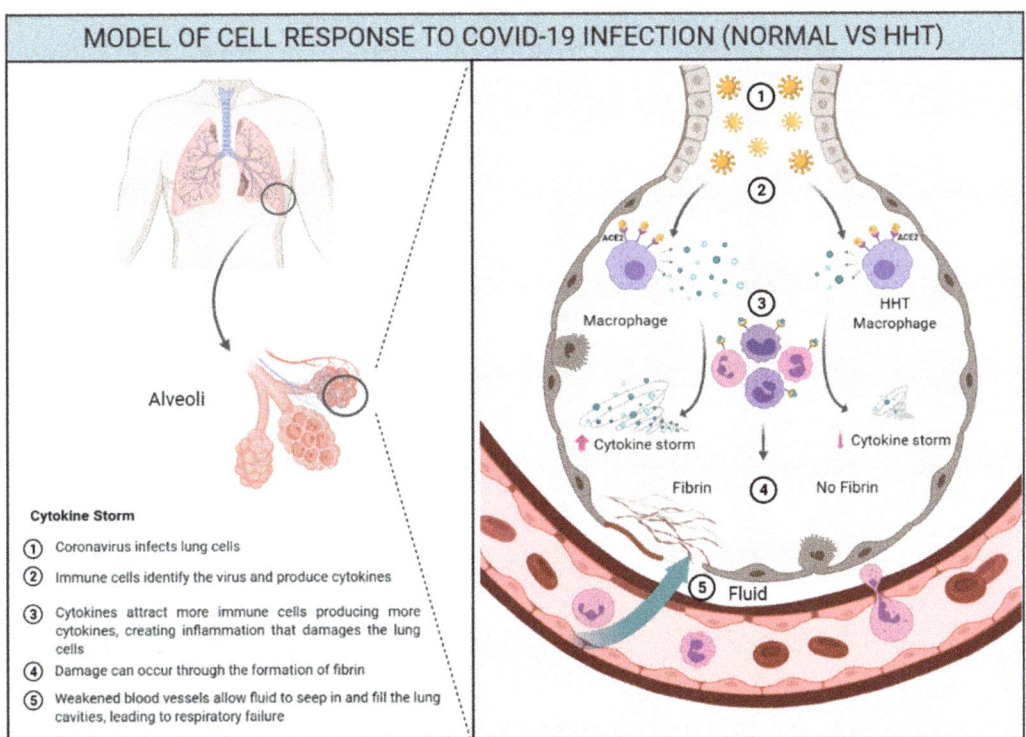

Figure 3. Graphical scheme explaining the COVID-19 reaction in HHT macrophages compared to macrophages of general population. The figure is based on the hypothesis that the cytokine production in HHT is not as exacerbated as the frequently occurred in the normal population leading to the "so-called" cytokine storm. 1. Coronavirus infects lung cells; 2. Immune cells, includes macrophages, identify the virus and produce cytokines; 3. Cytokines attract more immune cells, such as white blood cells, which in turn produce more cytokines, creating a cycle of inflammation that damages the lung cells; 4. Damage can occur through the formation of fibrin; 5. Weakened blood vessels allow fluid to seep in and fill the lung cavities, leading to respiratory failure.

Another disease where the HHT condition may confer a better outcome is cancer. In a mouse model of skin carcinoma, HHT mice developed fewer tumors then their wild type littermates. These studies suggest that endoglin behaved as a suppressor of malignancy in experimental and human epithelial carcinogenesis, although it could also promote metastasis in other types of cancer [30]. In humans, it has been hypothesized that individuals with HHT may be protected against life-limiting cancers [31] due to limited angiogenesis, since endoglin and ALK1 are proangiogenic factors. Anti-endoglin and anti-Alk1 therapies have been used for targeting tumors [32].

As a summary, the results of this communication suggest that HHT patients might be protected from developing a cytokine storm after SARS-CoV-2 infection. The results of this work represent, up to the moment, the largest series of HHT patients diagnosed of/affected by COVID-19 published to date. We are planning to conduct a larger survey with data derived from the HHT patient associations, at national and international levels, to gain more insights into HHT and the COVID-19 infection, and possibly reinforce this hypothesis.

Limitations and Interest of the Study

The main limitation of our study is that the sample analyzed represents a retrospective study of a group of patients belonging to a reference HHT ENT consult who attend regularly to this HCP, and not a random sample. Therefore, the results may not be representative for the whole HHT population, and the whole pandemic situation, but provide interesting interim results. The reason for focusing the survey on the patients attending the ENT consult is due to the fact that epistaxis is the most prevalent symptom in HHT, and moreover, this ENT consult is taking care of HHT patients from all over Spain, due to the degree of satisfaction of the HHT patients. Maybe the incidence of COVID-19 among these patients was even higher since not all received PCR testing. Asymptomatic COVID-19-positive patients could have been categorized as false negative.

We must realize that in rare diseases, the low prevalence of patients make this type of study difficult. We are aware that this is only a starting point to draw conclusions which may be confirmed by larger studies. On the other hand, this study presents the novelty of being a study conducted in an emergency situation. Perhaps it represents the first study where SARS-CoV-2 infection has been investigated in a cohort of patients with a rare disease.

Author Contributions: Conceptualization, S.M. and L.-M.B.; methodology, S.M., V.A., L.O.-F., B.T. and L.R.-P.; software, V.A, and L.O.-F.; validation, S.M., V.A., B.T., L.R.-P., M.P.V.-G., L.O.-F. and L.-M.B.; formal analysis, S.M., V.A. and B.T.; investigation, S.M., V.A. and L.O.-F.; resources, L.-M.B.; data curation, S.M.; writing—original draft preparation, L.-M.B.; writing—review and editing, V.A., L.O.-F. and L.-M.B.; visualization, S.M., V.A., B.T., L.R.-P., M.P.V.-G., L.O.-F. and L.-M.B.; supervision, V.A., L.O.-F. and L.-M.B.; project administration, L.-M.B.; funding acquisition, L.-M.B. All authors have read and agreed to the published version of the manuscript.

Funding: This research was funded by the Ministry of Economy and Competitivity MINECO, grant number SAF2017-83351R, and by a special internal project of CSIC (National Research Council of Spain) grant number PIE 201820E073. Additionally, V.A. is recipient of a grant from the Spanish Network of Research on Rare Diseases, CIBERER, unit 707.

Institutional Review Board Statement: The study was conducted according to the guidelines of the Declaration of Helsinki, and approved by the Ethics Committee of the National Research Council of Spain (CSIC), number 075-2017.

Informed Consent Statement: Informed consent was obtained from all subjects involved in the study, as well as from the patients to publish this paper.

Data Availability Statement: Reported results can be found in the files of Centro de Investigaciones Biológicas Margarita Salas (CIB, CSIC) and in the files of Hospital Universitario Fundación Alcorcón (HUFA), Madrid, Spain.

Acknowledgments: We acknowledge the HHT Spain Patient Association by their support and interest in this research, and in particular, to the patients who gave their consent and answered the questionnaire about the COVID-19 infection.

Conflicts of Interest: The authors declare no conflict of interest.

References

1. Ministerio de Sanidad, Consumo y Bienestar Social. Available online: https://www.mscbs.gob.es/profesionales/saludPublica/ccayes/alertasActual/nCov/situacionActual.htm (accessed on 23 March 2021).
2. Hamming, I.; Timens, W.; Bulthuis, M.L.; Lely, A.T.; Navis, G.; van Goor, H. Tissue distribution of ACE2 protein, the functional receptor for SARS coronavirus. A first step in understanding SARS pathogenesis. *J. Pathol.* **2004**, *203*, 6317. [CrossRef]
3. Ayres, J.S. A metabolic handbook for the COVID-19 pandemic. *Nat. Metab.* **2020**, *2*, 572–585. [CrossRef]
4. Teuwen, L.A.; Geldhof, V.; Pasut, A.; Carmeliet, P. COVID-19: The vasculature unleashed. *Nat. Rev. Immunol.* **2020**, *20*, 389–391. [CrossRef] [PubMed]
5. Shovlin, C.L.; Guttmacher, A.E.; Buscarini, E.; Faughnan, M.E.; Hyland, R.H.; Westermann, C.J.J.; Kjeldsen, A.D.; Plauchu, H. Diagnostic criteria for Hereditary Hemorrhagic Telangiectasia (Rendu-Osler-Weber Syndrome). *Am. J. Med. Genet.* **2000**, *91*, 66–67. [CrossRef]
6. Shovlin, C.L. Hereditary haemorrhagic telangiectasia: Pathophysiology, diagnosis and treatment. *Blood Rev.* **2010**, *24*, 203–219. [CrossRef] [PubMed]
7. Shovlin, C.L. Pulmonary arteriovenous malformations. *Am. J. Respir. Crit. Care Med.* **2014**, *190*, 1217–1228. [CrossRef]

8. Kjeldsen, A.D.; Vase, P.; Green, A. Hereditary haemorrhagic telangiectasia: A population-based study of prevalence and mortality in Danish patients. *J. Intern. Med.* **1999**, *245*, 31–39. [CrossRef] [PubMed]
9. Jessurun, G.A.J.; Kamphuis, D.J.; van der Zande, F.H.R.; Nossent, J.C. Cerebral arteriovenous malformations in the Netherlands Antilles. High prevalence of hereditary hemorrhagic telangiectasia-related single and multiple cerebral arteriovenous malformations. *Clin. Neurol. Neurosurg.* **1993**, *95*, 193–198. [CrossRef]
10. McAllister, K.A.; Grogg, K.M.; Johnson, D.W.; Gallione, C.J.; Baldwin, M.A.; Jackson, C.E.; Helmbold, E.A.; Markel, D.S.; McKinnon, W.C.; Murrel, J.; et al. Endoglin, a TGF-β binding protein of endothelial cells, is the gene for hereditary haemorrhagic telangiectasia type 1. *Nat. Genet.* **1994**, *8*, 345–351. [CrossRef]
11. Johnson, D.W.; Berg, J.N.; Baldwin, M.A.; Gallione, C.J.; Marondel, I.; Yoon, S.J.; Stenzel, T.T.; Speer, M.; Pericak-Vance, M.A.; Diamond, A.; et al. Mutations in the activin receptor-like kinase 1 gene in hereditary haemorrhagic telangiectasia type. *Nat. Genet.* **1996**, *13*, 189–195. [CrossRef]
12. Morales-Angulo, C.; Del Valle-Zapico, A. Hereditary hemorrhagic telangiectasia. *Otolaryngol. Head Neck Surg.* **1998**, *119*, 293.
13. Assar, O.S.; Friedman, C.M.; White, R.I. The Natural History of Epistaxis in Hereditary Hemorrhagic Telangiectasia. *Laryngoscope* **1991**, *101*, 977–980. [CrossRef]
14. Geisthoff, U.W.; Schneider, G.; Fischinger, J.; Plinkert, P.K. Hereditary hemorrhagic telangiectasia (Osler's disease). An interdisciplinary challenge. *HNO* **2002**, *50*, 114–128. [CrossRef]
15. Guttmacher, A.E.; Marchuk, D.A.; White, R.I. Hereditary hemorrhagic telangiectasia. *N. Engl. J. Med.* **1995**, *333*, 918–924. [CrossRef]
16. Esteban-Casado, S.; Martín de Rosales Cabrera, A.M.; Usarral de Pérez, A.; Martínez Simón, J.J.; Zhan Zhou, E.; Marcos Salazar, M.S.; Pérez Encinas, M.; Botella Cubells, L. Sclerotherapy and Topical Nasal Propranolol: An Effective and Safe Therapy for HHT-Epistaxis. *Laryngoscope* **2019**, *129*, 2216–2223. [CrossRef]
17. Sánchez-Martínez, R.; Iriarte, A.; Mora-Luján, J.M.; Patier, J.L.; López-Wolf, D.; Ojeda, A.; Torralba, M.A.; Juyol, M.C.; Gil, R.; Añón, S.; et al. RiHHTa Investigators of the Rare Diseases Working Group from the Spanish Society of Internal Medicine. Current HHT genetic overview in Spain and its phenotypic correlation: Data from RiHHTa registry. *Orphanet J. Rare Dis.* **2020**, *15*, 138. [CrossRef]
18. Fernandez-L, A.; Sanz-Rodriguez, F.; Zarrabeitia, R.; Perez-Molino, A.; Morales, C.; Restrepo, C.M.; Ramirez, J.R.; Coto, E.; Lenato, G.M.; Bernabeu, C.; et al. Mutation study of spanish patients with hereditary hemorrhagic telangiectasia and expression analysis of endoglin and ALK1. *Hum. Mutat.* **2006**, *27*, 295. [CrossRef]
19. Health National Institute Carlos III. Report No. 70, COVID-19 Situation in Spain. Available online: https://www.isciii.es/QueHacemos/Servicios/VigilanciaSaludPublicaRENAVE/EnfermedadesTransmisibles/Documents/INFORMES/Informes%20COVID-19/INFORMES%20COVID-19%202021/Informe%20COVID-19.%20N%C2%BA%2070_%2017%20de%20marzo%20de%202021.pdf (accessed on 17 March 2021).
20. Sierra-Filardi, E.; Puig-Kröger, A.; Blanco, F.J.; Nieto, C.; Bragado, R.; Palomero, M.I.; Bernabéu, C.; Vega, M.A.; Corbí, A.L. Activin A skews macrophage polarization by promoting a proinflammatory phenotype and inhibiting the acquisition of anti-inflammatory macrophage markers. *Blood* **2011**, *117*, 5092–5101. [CrossRef]
21. Nalbandian, A.; Sehgal, K.; Gupta, A.; Madhavan, M.V.; McGroder, C.; Stevens, J.S.; Cook, J.R.; Nordvig, A.S.; Shalev, D.; Sehrawat, T.S.; et al. Post-acute COVID-19 syndrome. *Nat. Med.* **2021**, in press. [CrossRef]
22. Riera-Mestre, A.; Iriarte, A.; Moreno, M.; del Castillo, R.; López-Wolf, D. Angiogenesis, hereditary hemorrhagic telangiectasia and COVID-19. *Angiogenesis* **2021**, *24*, 13–15. [CrossRef]
23. Zhou, P.; Yang, X.L.; Wang, X.G.; Hu, B.; Zhang, L.; Zhang, W.; Si, H.R.; Zhu, Y.; Li, B.; Huang, C.L.; et al. A pneumonia outbreak associated with a new coronavirus of probable bat origin. *Nature* **2020**, *579*, 270–273. [CrossRef]
24. Alijotas-Reig, J.; Esteve-Valverde, E.; Belizna, C.; Selva-O'Callaghan, A.; Pardos-Gea, J.; Quintana, A.; Mekinian, A.; Anunciacion-Llunell, A.; Miró-Mur, F. Immunomodulatory therapy for the management of severe COVID-19. Beyond the anti-viral therapy: A comprehensive review. *Autoimmun. Rev.* **2020**, *19*, 102569. [CrossRef]
25. WHO Solidarity Trial Consortium; Pan, H.; Peto, R.; Henao-Restrepo, A.-M.; Preziosi, M.-P.; Sathiyamoorthy, V.; Abdool Karim, Q.; Alejandria, M.M.; Hernández García, C.; Kieny, M.-P.; et al. Repurposed Antiviral Drugs for COVID-19—Interim WHO Solidarity Trial Results. *N. Engl. J. Med.* **2021**, *384*, 497–511.
26. Moffat, J.G.; Vincent, F.; Lee, J.A.; Eder, J.; Prunotto, M. Opportunities and challenges in phenotypic drug discovery: An industry perspective. *Nat. Rev. Drug Discov.* **2017**, *16*, 531–543. [CrossRef]
27. RECOVERY Collaborative Group; Horby, P.; Lim, W.S.; Emberson, J.R.; Mafham, M.; Bell, J.L.; Linsell, L.; Staplin, N.; Brightling, C.; Ustianowski, A.; et al. Dexamethasone in Hospitalized Patients with COVID-19. *N. Engl. J. Med.* **2021**, *384*, 693–704.
28. Zhou, F.; Yu, T.; Du, R.; Fan, G.; Liu, Y.; Liu, Z.; Xiang, J.; Wang, Y.; Song, B.; Gu, X.; et al. Clinical course and risk factors for mortality of adult inpatients with COVID-19 in Wuhan, China: A retrospective cohort study. *Lancet* **2020**, *395*, 1054–1062. [CrossRef]
29. Ojeda-Fernández, L.; Recio-Poveda, L.; Aristorena, M.; Lastres, P.; Blanco, F.J.; Sanz-Rodríguez, F.; Gallardo-Vara, E.; de las Casas-Engel, M.; Corbí, Á.; Arthur, H.M.; et al. Mice Lacking Endoglin in Macrophages Show an Impaired Immune Response. *PLoS Genet.* **2016**, *12*, e1005935. [CrossRef]
30. Pérez-Gómez, E.; Del Castillo, G.; Juan Francisco, S.; López-Novoa, J.M.; Bernabéu, C.; Quintanilla, M. The role of the TGF-β coreceptor endoglin in cancer. *Sci. World J.* **2010**, *10*, 2367–2384. [CrossRef]

31. Hosman, A.E.; Devlin, H.L.; Silva, B.M.; Shovlin, C.L. Specific cancer rates may differ in patients with hereditary haemorrhagic telangiectasia compared to controls. *Orphanet J. Rare Dis.* **2013**, *8*, 195. [CrossRef]
32. Toi, H.; Tsujie, M.; Haruta, Y.; Fujita, K.; Duzen, J.; Seon, B.K. Facilitation of endoglin-targeting cancer therapy by development/utilization of a novel genetically engineered mouse model expressing humanized endoglin (CD105). *Int. J. Cancer* **2015**, *136*, 452–461. [CrossRef]

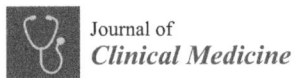 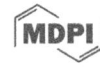

Review

Founder Effects in Hereditary Hemorrhagic Telangiectasia

Tamás Major [1,*], Réka Gindele [2], Gábor Balogh [2], Péter Bárdossy [3] and Zsuzsanna Bereczky [2,*]

1. Division of Otorhinolaryngology and Head & Neck Surgery, Kenézy Gyula Campus, University of Debrecen Medical Center, H-4031 Debrecen, Hungary
2. Division of Clinical Laboratory Science, Department of Laboratory Medicine, Faculty of Medicine, University of Debrecen, H-4032 Debrecen, Hungary; gindele.reka@med.unideb.hu (R.G.); balogh.gabor@med.unideb.hu (G.B.)
3. Hungarian Heraldry and Genealogical Society, H-1014 Budapest, Hungary; peter@bardossy.hu
* Correspondence: major.tamas@kenezy.unideb.hu (T.M.); zsbereczky@med.unideb.hu (Z.B.); Tel.: +36-52-511777/1756 (T.M.); +36-52-431956 (Z.B.); Fax: +36-52-511755 (T.M.); +36-52-340011 (Z.B.)

Abstract: A founder effect can result from the establishment of a new population by individuals from a larger population or bottleneck events. Certain alleles may be found at much higher frequencies because of genetic drift immediately after the founder event. We provide a systematic literature review of the sporadically reported founder effects in hereditary hemorrhagic telangiectasia (HHT). All publications from the *ACVRL1*, *ENG* and *SMAD4* Mutation Databases and publications searched for terms "hereditary hemorrhagic telangiectasia" and "founder" in PubMed and Scopus, respectively, were extracted. Following duplicate removal, 141 publications were searched for the terms "founder" and "founding" and the etymon "ancest". Finally, 67 publications between 1992 and 2020 were reviewed. Founder effects were graded upon shared area of ancestry/residence, shared core haplotypes, genealogy and prevalence. Twenty-six *ACVRL1* and 12 *ENG* variants with a potential founder effect were identified. The bigger the cluster of families with a founder mutation, the more remarkable is its influence to the populational *ACVRL1/ENG* ratio, affecting HHT phenotype. Being aware of founder effects might simplify the diagnosis of HHT by establishing local genetic algorithms. Families sharing a common core haplotype might serve as a basis to study potential second-hits in the etiology of HHT.

Keywords: hereditary hemorrhagic telangiectasia; germline mutation; founder effect; haplotype; genealogy; population genetics

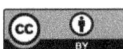

1. Introduction

1.1. Definition

A founder effect may result from the establishment of a new population by individuals deriving from a much larger population (a true founder event) or an extreme reduction in population size (a bottleneck event). As a consequence, certain alleles may be found at a higher frequency than previously and can reach even a higher prevalence by genetic drift in the period immediately after the founder event, and later, by inbreeding, particularly in population isolates [1].

1.2. Founder Effects in Population Isolates

Population isolates serve as an excellent basis for the investigation of founder effects. They exist in isolation from other populations as a result of cultural (linguistic or religious) or geographical (mountains, seas, deserts, etc.) barriers [2]. The best-known cultural population isolates are the Ashkenazi Jews and North American Anabaptist groups (the Mennonites, the Hutterites and the Old Order Amish). Each of these is characterized by little genetic inflow, identifiable small founding population and well-known historical bottleneck events, high standard of living, high interest in illness and highly accessible medical care [3,4]. The Anabaptist communities, furthermore, keep extensive genealogical records, live in large families with low rates of non-paternity and high rates of consanguinity and have notably uniform socioeconomic circumstances [3,5].

As a result of founder effects, both the cultural and geographical population isolates have their characteristic Mendelian (autosomal recessive, autosomal dominant and X-linked) or mitochondrial disorders. The increased incidence of these otherwise rare conditions allows for linkage analysis and identification of causative genes [3,6]. Founder alleles might contribute to the risk for more common complex diseases, like type II diabetes, obesity or bipolar affective illness in the Mennonites and Amish [5,7]. Moreover, several population isolates exhibit peculiar founder germline dominant *BRCA1/2* alleles with early onset breast and ovarian cancer risks [4,8,9]. Consequently, population isolate-specific databases and screening panels for genetic disorders might be established [4,10].

1.3. Pioneer Reports for Founder Effects in Hereditary Hemorrhagic Telangiectasia

The majority of familial (germline) vascular malformations or syndromes are inherited in an autosomal dominant trait and mutations are usually family specific [11]. Although, per definitionem, it is considered to be a rare disease (with a prevalence beneath 1 in 2000) [12], hereditary hemorrhagic telangiectasia (HHT) is the most common inherited arteriovenous malformation syndrome [11]. The so-far identified causative genes are *ENG* and *ACVRL1* (accounting for HHT1 and HHT2, respectively, over 85% of all HHT cases), *SMAD4* (JP/HHT phenotype, 2% of HHT cases) and *GDF2* (HHT5, reported occasionally) [13]. The worldwide prevalence of HHT is 1:5000–1:10,000 [14]. However, this widely accepted value is an estimate. Prior to the identification of *ENG* and *ACVRL1* in the mid-nineties [15,16], direct questionnaire (addressed to general practitioners and specialists) and/or hospital record-based methods were performed to assess the prevalence of HHT, with variable return rates and results (2.5–19.4 per 100,000) [17–21]. Each author highlighted that these results were underestimates. Despite the variable prevalence rates, population genetic studies reported some geographical regions with prominently high point-prevalences, like Ain, Jura and Deux-Sevres Counties of France or the islands of Curacao and Bonaire of the Netherlands Antilles [18,22]. Subsequent comprehensive molecular genetic studies showed unrelated families within these areas with identical *ENG* and *ACVRL1* mutations and shared adjacent core haplotypes, suggesting common ancestry [23–25]. If one or few of these variants with common ancestry dominate a geographic area, its founder effect is confirmed.

In the present study, we provide a systematic literature review of founder effects in HHT, reported in the past two decades.

2. Study Design

2.1. Literature Search

The targets of the literature search were (1) all publications referred in the *ENG*, *ACVRL1* and *SMAD4* Databases, respectively [26–28]; (2) results from PubMed and Scopus for *"hereditary hemorrhagic telangiectasia" (all fields)* AND *"founder" (all fields)* (both databases were accessed on 9 February 2021). Following the removal of papers considered as irrelevant based on their abstracts and duplicates from the primary pool, the whole text of 141 publications was subsequently searched for the terms *"founder"* and *"founding"* and the etymon *"ancest"*. The resulting 67 papers (listed in Supplementary Materials Table S1) and if required, their references were independently searched for HHT founder mutations by the authors T.M. and R.G. (Figure 1).

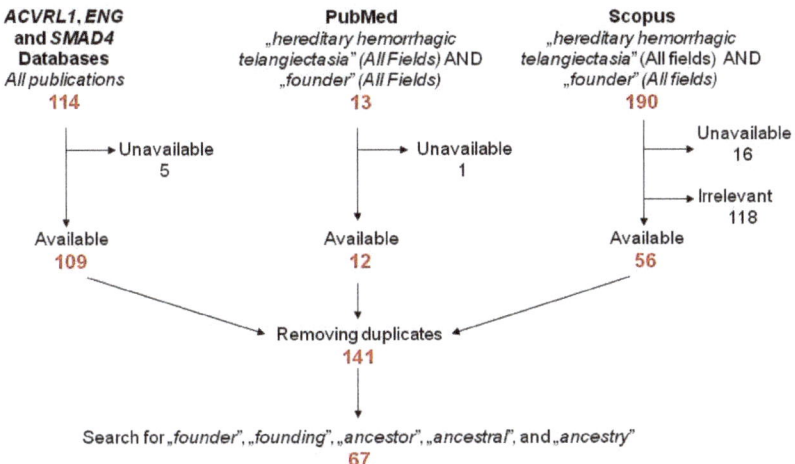

Figure 1. The algorithm of the literature search for hereditary hemorrhagic telangiectasia (HHT) founder effects.

2.2. An Arbitrary Grading System to Assess Evidences for Founder Effect in HHT

In the aforementioned areas with elevated HHT point-prevalence, geographical barriers (island or mountains) are suspected. However, in the midst of expanding transport potentials in the 20th and the 21st century the significance of geographical barriers as the main reason for population isolates is declining. On the other hand, HHT is not detected in known cultural population isolates. Therefore, we assume that the magnitude of a founder effect in HHT is also continuously declining even in previous geographical population isolates, essentially by emigration and immigration [25]. By reviewing the literature, pieces of evidence for founder effects were collected as follows: (1) if identical causative mutations are detected in unrelated families by a laboratory with expertise in HHT genetics; (2) if families with an identical mutation originate from or live in the same geographical area; (3) if there is genealogical evidence of common ancestry; (4) if shared core haplotypes are detected by intragenic and flanking extragenic polymorphic markers; and (5) if the investigated mutation is still prevalent in the given geographical area, thus responsible for the majority of causative variants. The simultaneous reports of shared core haplotype and shared area of ancestry/residence as pieces of evidence for a founder effect were especially frequent.

Somewhat arbitrarily, we constructed a grading system to assess founder effects in HHT (Table 1). Criteria were weighted by the number of kindreds reported. The terms "apparently unrelated families", "shared area of ancestry or residence", "shared core haplotype" and "genealogical evidence of common ancestry" were not uniformly and unequivocally defined in the majority of papers. In these cases, we accepted the authors' self-report. Although a core haplotype shared by a few (2–4) families only, refers to their potential common ancestor, from a population genetic point of view; however, it is not strong enough to prove the founder effect. If these families still live in or originate from the same area, it might be a stronger argument at the founder effect. Unrelated families were defined only in two papers, as "not related by blood within living memory" [22], or "unrelated going back for at least four generations" [29]. Here we define a mutation as "locally still prevalent", if it accounts for $\geq 30\%$ of all HHT families or cases in an administrative area (minimum a district of a county) or distorts national HHT mutation distribution by presenting in a $\geq 10\%$ proportion.

Table 1. Our grading system to assess evidences for founder effects in HHT.

Grade	Description
I	Identical mutation in apparently unrelated families in a HHT center
II	Shared area of ancestry/residence (2–4) OR Shared core haplotype (2–4) OR Genealogical evidence of common ancestry (2–4)
III	Shared area of ancestry/residence ($\geq$5) OR Shared core haplotype ($\geq$5) OR Genealogical evidence of common ancestry ($\geq$5) OR shared core haplotype (2–4) AND shared area of ancestry/residence (2–4)
IV	Grade 3 AND a locally still-prevalent mutation

Numbers in parentheses refer to the number of families.

If a variant fulfilled the criteria of a minimum grade II founder effect in any of the publications, it was collected, even the absence of authors' self-report as a founder. Furthermore, all other available reports of the captured minimum grade II founders were reviewed.

At the assessment of mutation pathogenicity, we accepted authors' self-report. In the case of variants indicated as "pending" in the *ENG* and *ACVRL1* Databases [26,27], we reassessed variant pathogenicity by in silico prediction analyses and authors' arguments (co-segregation, absence in healthy controls, comparison with ortologs, etc.) (Supplementary Materials Table S2). At variant classification, we followed the joint consensus recommendations of the American College of Medical Genetics and Genomics (ACMG) [30].

3. The Overview of Potential Founders

3.1. Variant Distribution, Type and Pathogenicity

A total of 26 *ACVRL1* and 12 *ENG* variants (Table 2) were identified with grade I to IV founder effects. The *ACVRL1* c.1445C>T variant was assessed as benign and excluded from further analysis.

Table 2. Grade I to IV founder variants in the *ACVRL1* and *ENG* genes.

Location	ACVRL1 Variant	Type	Classification	Population	No. of Families	Founder Grade	Comment	Reference	Independent Reference
Ex 3	c.152G>A, p.Cys51Tyr	M	P	Italian (Pavia—Crema Center)	2	II	Shared area of ancestry	[29]	[31,32]
	c.199C>T, p.Arg67Trp	M	P	Italian (Pavia—Crema Center)	2	III	Shared haplotype AND area of ancestry	[33]	[34–37]
				Italian (Pavia—Crema Center)	2	II	Shared area of ancestry	[29]	
				German	2	I	Recurrent	[35]	
		M	P	French and Italian	3	II	Shared haplotype 1	[25]	
				French	2	II	Shared haplotype 2	[25]	
	c.200G>A, p.Arg67Gln			Italian (Pavia—Crema Center)	3	II	Shared area of ancestry	[29]	[38,39]
				Italian (Bari Center)	4	I	Recurrent	[31] [40]	
					3	I	Recurrent		
				Han Chinese	2	I	Recurrent	[41]	
	c.205_209dupTGCGG p.Asn71Alafs*53	FS	P	Italian	2	II	Shared area of ancestry	[29]	
	c.265 T>C, p.Cys89Arg	M	LP	Hungarian (Nógrád County)	3	II [2]	Genealogy	[42]	
	289-294delCACAAC p.His97_Asn98del	D	LP [1]	Italian (Pavia—Crema Center)	2	III	Shared haplotype AND area of ancestry	[33]	
				Italian (Bergamo County)	10	III-IV [2]	Shared area of residence. Prevalent? [4]	[29]	
Ex 4	c.430C>T, p.Arg144*	N	P	French	2	II	Shared haplotype	[24]	[31,41,43–45]
				French and Italian	7	III [2]	Shared haplotype. Age estimate: 22 gen	[25]	
				Italian	4	I	Recurrent	[29]	
Int 5	c.625+1G>C	SS	P	Hungarian (Heves County)	7	IV [2]	Shared area of residence, shared haplotype, genealogy, prevalent [4]	[46,47]	
Ex 6	c.651G>A, p.Trp217*	N	P	Norwegian (Østfold County and West Sweden)	7	IV [2]	Shared area of ancestry, shared haplotype, prevalent [4]	[48]	[49]

107

Table 2. Cont.

Location	ACVRL1 Variant	Type	Classi-Fication	Population	No. of Families	Founder Grade	Comment	Reference	Independent Reference
Ex 7	c.830C>A, p.Thr277Lys	M	P	Norwegian (Rana, Nordland County)	13	IV [2]	Shared area of ancestry, shared haplotype, prevalent [4]	[48]	
	c.924C>A, p.Cys308*	N	P	Italian (Pavia–Crema Center)	2	II	Shared area of ancestry	[29]	[38,40]
	c.998G>T, p.Ser333Ile	M	P	American (Utah, US) American (Toronto Center)	5 +1	III-IV	Genealogy. Prevalent? [4] Area of ancestry in Utah, US [4]	[50] [43,51]	[40]
	c.1042delG, p.Asp348Thrfs*6	FS	P	Dutch	7	III [2]	Genealogy in 5 families [4]	[52]	
Ex 8	c.1055C>A, p.Ala352Asp	M	P	American (Massachusetts, US)	2	II [2]	Shared haplotype	[53]	

Location	ACVRL1 Variant	Type	Classi-Fication	Population	No. of Families	Founder Grade	Comment	Reference	Independent Reference
Ex 8	c.1112_1113dupG p.Thr372Hisfs*20	FS	P	French (Valserine Valley, Jura County)	17	IV [2]	Shared area of ancestry/residence, shared haplotype, prevalent [4]	[24]	
				French	35	IV [2]	Shared area of ancestry/residence, shared haplotype, prevalent. Age estimate: 13 gen [4]	[25]	
				European and North American	+1?		Area of ancestry in the Rhône-Alpes region, France [4]	[51]	
				American (Utah, US)	+1		Area of ancestry in Ain, France [4]	[54]	
	c.1120C>T, p.Arg374Trp	M	P	French and Italian	6	III [2]	Shared haplotype. Age estimate: 11 gen [4]	[25]	[35,40,55–58]
				American (Ontario, Canada)	2	I	Recurrent	[34,43]	
				Dutch	3	I	Recurrent	[52]	
				American	2	I	Recurrent	[54]	
				Italian (Bari Center)	2	I	Recurrent	[38]	
				Italian (Pavia–Crema Center)	3	II	Shared area of ancestry	[29]	
				Han Chinese	2	I [3]	Recurrent	[39]	

Table 2. Cont.

Location	ACVRL1 Variant	Type	Classi-Fication	Population	No. of Families	Founder Grade	Comment	Reference	Independent Reference
	c.1121G>A, p.Arg374Gln	M	P	French (Deux-Sèvres County)	3	III [2]	Shared haplotype 1 AND area of ancestry [4]	[25]	[29,37,56,59,60]
				European and North American	+3?	II	Shared area of ancestry in Parthenay, Deux-Sèvres County, France. Age estimate: 4 gen [4]	[51]	
				French (Northeast France)	3	III [2]	Shared haplotype 2 AND area of ancestry [4]	[25]	
	c.1126A>G, p.Met376Val	M	P	French	3	II	Shared haplotype	[25]	[59]
	c.1199C>A, p.Ala400Asp	M	P	Italian (Pavia–Crema Center)	2	II	Shared area of ancestry	[29]	
	c.1231C>T, p.Arg411Trp	M	P	French	7	III [2]	Shared haplotype	[24]	[35,61]
					9	III [2]	Shared haplotype. Age estimate: 15 gen	[25]	
				American (Ontario, Canada)	2	I	Recurrent	[34]	
				Dutch	2	I	Recurrent	[52]	
				German	3	I	Recurrent	[41]	
	c.1232G>A, p.Arg411Gln	M	P	North American	2	II	Shared area of ancestry	[51]	[38,40,56,60,62]
				French	2	II	Shared haplotype	[25]	
				American (Utah, US)	2	I	Recurrent	[54]	
				Italian (Pavia–Crema Center)	2	II	Shared area of ancestry	[29]	
				Han Chinese	3	I [3]	Recurrent	[39]	
	c.1232G>C, p.Arg411Pro	M	P	French	2	II	Shared haplotype	[24]	[59]
Location	ACVRL1 Variant	Type	Classi-Fication	Population	No. of Families	Founder Grade	Comment	Reference	Independent Reference
Ex 9	c.1280A>T, p.Asp427Val	M	P [1]	French	2	II	Shared haplotype	[25]	[38]
Int 9	c.1377+2T>A	SS	LP	Hungarian (Heves and Borsod Counties)	2	II	Genealogy	[42]	

Table 2. Cont.

Location	ACVRL1 Variant	Type	Classi-Fication	Population	No. of Families	Founder Grade	Comment	Reference	Independent Reference
Ex 10	c.1435C>T, p.Arg479*	N	P	French	2	II	Shared haplotype	[24]	[29,37,38,52, 59,60,63,64]
					2	II	Shared haplotype	[25]	
				Japanese (West Japan)	2	I	Recurrent	[45]	
	c.1450C>T, p.Arg484Trp	M	P	Norwegian (Nordland County)	5	III-IV [2]	Shared haplotype. Prevalent? [4]	[48]	[25,29,52, 61]
				Italian (Bari Center)	2	I	Recurrent	[38]	

Location	ENG Variant	Type	Classi-Fication	Population	No. of Families	Founder Grade	Comment	Reference	Independent Reference
Int 1	c.67+1G>A	SS	P	Netherlands Antillean Dutch	7 +1	IV [2]	Shared haplotype, prevalent [4]	[23] [52]	
Ex 3	c.277C>T, p.Arg93*	N	P	Italian	3	II	Shared area of ancestry	[29]	[44,52,59, 65]
				Norwegian (Southeast)	5	I	Recurrent. Haplotype analysis showed different haplotypes [4]	[48]	
	c.360C>A, p.Tyr120*	N	P	Danish (Funen County)	7	IV [2]	shared haplotype, shared area of residence, prevalent. Age estimate: 13–14 gen [4]	[44]	
				Danish (Funen county)	7	IV [2]	Shared area of residence, prevalent [4]	[66]	
				Danish (Nationwide)	13	IV [2]	Shared area of residence, prevalent [4]	[67]	
Int 3	c.360+1G>A	SS	P	Italian (Pavia–Crema Center)	2	II	Shared area of ancestry	[29]	[41,52,54,68, 69]
Ex 6	c.781T>C, p.Trp261Arg	M	P [1]	Dutch	8	II	Genealogy in 3 families [4]	[52]	
Int 6	c.817-2 A>C	SS	P	Hungarian (Heves and Borsod Counties)	2	II [2]	Shared area of ancestry, genealogy [4]	[42]	
Ex 7	c.828_829insA, p.Tyr277Ilefs*57	FS	P	Japanese (Akita, County A, Japan)	2	III-IV [2]	Shared haplotype AND area of residence. Prevalent? [4]	[70]	
Int 7	c.1134+1G>A	SS	P	English (South England)	2	III	Shared haplotype AND area of residence	[71]	

Table 2. *Cont.*

Location	*ACVRL1* Variant	Type	Classi-fication	Population	No. of Families	Founder Grade	Comment	Reference	Independent Reference
Ex 9	c.1238G>T, p.Gly413Val	M	P [1]	Netherlands Antillean and Dutch Dutch	3 +1?	**III** [2]	Shared haplotype AND area of ancestry [4]	[23] [52]	
Int 10	c.1311G>A, p.Arg437Arg	SS	VUS [1]	Dutch	5	**III** [2]	Genealogy [4]	[52]	
Ex 12	c.1630delA, p.Thr544Profs*8	FS	P	American (Ontario, Canada)	2	**II**	Shared area of ancestry	[34]	
Int 12	c.1686+5G>C	SS	LP [1]	Spanish	3	**I** [3]	Recurrent	[60]	

Abbreviations and legends: At the intragenic location, Ex = exon and Int = intron. At the variant location, D = in-frame deletion, FS = frameshift, M = missense, N = nonsense and SS = splice-site. At the pathogenicity classification (Classification), P = pathogenic, LP = likely pathogenic, VUS = variant of uncertain significance. [1] Pathogenicity of a pending variant is reassessed (Supplementary Materials Table S2). [2] variant reported as a founder; [3] variant reported as a founder or a hot-spot. Bolds: the highest founder grade of a variant reported by a given research group. At the comment, gen = generation; [4] detailed in the text. Independent Reference: report of the variant by independent authors (if a research group reported the variant several times, the first report is given).

Neither the *SMAD4* variants associated with the HHT or JP/HHT phenotype nor the extremely rare *GDF2* were reported as founders [72,73].

The distribution of founders throughout the *ACVRL1* and the *ENG* genes is similar to all mutations available in the databases [26,27]. The majority (16/26) of *ACVRL1* founder variants (Figure 2) is missense type, clustering within exons 3 and 8. Missense variants in exon 3 of the extracellular domain might impair TGF-β receptor type I and II interactions and ligand-dependent signaling [43]. Missense variants in exon 8 involve highly conserved amino acids (c.1120C>T and c.1121G>A affect Arg in codon 374, while c.1231C>T, c.1232G>C and c.1232G>A affect Arg in codon 411) within the core of the intracellular kinase C-lobe, compared to ortologs and paralogs [24,39,43,48,52,54]. Codons 374 and 411 are considered as mutation hot-spots, but several of them appear as grade II or even grade III founders in distinct geographical areas (Table 2) [24,25]. Interestingly, all but three of the variants (88.5%) were pathogenic, substantially exceeding the 64.5% given in the *ACVRL1* Database [27].

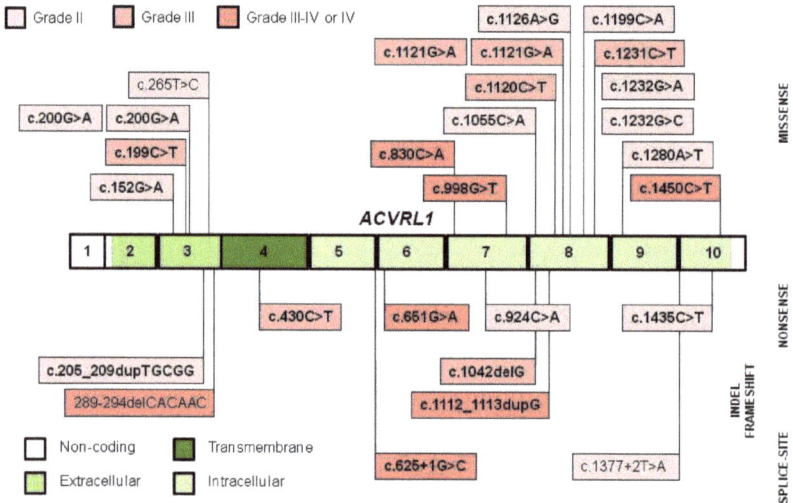

Figure 2. The grade II to IV founder variants in the exons and flanking intronic regions of *ACVRL1*. Pathogenic variants are indicated in bold. In the case of the c.200G>A and the c.1121G>A variants, two distinct flanking haplotypes were identified [25].

Founder *ENG* variants (Figure 3) tend to localize throughout its exons encoding the extracellular domain, with more nonsense, frameshift and splice-site and less missense variants [24,43,48,54,67]. Ten out of the 12 variants (83.3%) are pathogenic, similarly to the 78.9% given in the *ENG* Database [26].

Although founder effects and hot-spots are not excluding terms, we suppose that max. grade II variants with several independent reports (the *AVCRL1* c.152G>A, c.200G>A, c.924C>A, c.1232G>A and c.1435C>T; and the *ENG* c.277C>T and c.360+1G>A in Table 2), are rather hot-spots than founders and accordingly, were not considered as founder variants by the authors, either. Grade III or IV variants with several independent reports (the *ACVRL1* c.199C>T, c.430C>T, c.1120C>T, c.1121G>A, c.1231C>T and c.1450C>T in Table 2) might be hot-spots with local founder effects, in agreement with the authors.

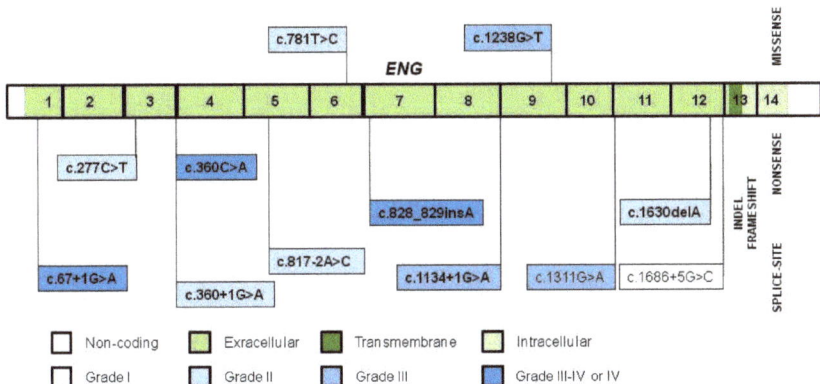

Figure 3. The grade II to IV founder variants in the exons and flanking intronic regions of *ENG*. Pathogenic variants are indicated in bold.

3.2. Grade IV Founder Variants

Henceforth, we focus on the *ACVRL1* and *ENG* variants with unequivocal founder effects.

We detected an identical *ACVRL1* c.625+1G>C pathogenic splice-site mutation in 19 individuals of five unrelated families in Heves County, Hungary [46]. Neither the probands nor their available alive kinships were acquainted with the others. Haplotype analysis with a total of eight intragenic and flanking extragenic polymorphic markers showed correspondent haplotypes at the tested region of the mutant chromosome. Subsequent genealogical analysis revealed a marriage from 1779 as the potential common ancestor of families. According to our stratified population screening study performed in order to assess HHT point-prevalence in the primary attendance area of the Ferenc Markhot County Hospital, Eger, Hungary (population of 225,000 in May 2017), this mutation dominated the study area by 57.7% (15/26 HHT patients) [47]. Currently, 21 tested heterozygous individuals of seven families constitute this kindred, still with a correspondent core haplotype (Supplementary Materials Figure S1). A non-complete geographical isolation given by the underdeveloped road network and the very low standard of living up to the beginning of the 20th century is considerable.

The *ACVRL1* c.651G>A pathogenic nonsense variant was detected in 26 patients of seven families from Østfold (Southeastern Norway) and neighboring West Sweden. Haplotype analysis was performed in five of these families, showing a common core haplotype [48]. From a nationwide point of view, this mutation accounts for 6.2% (6/113) of all and 7.2% (7/97) mutation positive HHT families and 11.1% (26/234) of HHT patients in Norway.

The *ACVRL1* c.830C>A (p.Thr277Lys) pathogenic missense variant was detected in 24 Norwegian families, with 22 of them originating from Rana District in Nordland County. Haplotype analysis was performed in 13/24 families, showing a shared core haplotype. This mutation dominates HHT in this geographical area, and furthermore, accounts for 21.2% (24/113) of all HHT families, and additionally, 24.7% (24/97) of HHT families and 24.8% (58/234) of HHT patients with an identified pathogenic or likely pathogenic mutation in Norway [48]. The area's localization in the proximity of the Arctic Circle and its landscape consisted of fjords and mountains might have served as potential causes of a past geographical isolation.

The *ACVRL1* c.1112_1113dupG pathogenic frameshift variant was initially described in 2003, by Abdalla et al., in 8 of 15 individuals of a family originating from the Rhône-Alpes region, France [43,51]. One year later, Lesca et al. reported this variant in 17 unrelated index cases [24], collected through the French HHT network. In microsatellite studies all patients shared a common haplotype. At that time, this variant accounted for 17% (17/100) of all identified family-specific HHT mutations, appreciably skewing the nationwide *ACVRL1/ENG* ratio. By 2008, already 35 families were known with this variant, still with a common core haplotype and an estimated age of the most recent common ancestor of 325 years. Although not exclusive in the area, this mutation is dominating HHT in Ain and Jura of the Rhône-Alpes region, with its epicenter to the Valserine valley [22,25]. The authors speculate that the founder event might have occurred in this region, prior to the 17th, century either as a de novo variant or by immigration, and subsequently, it increased in prevalence due to genetic drift in the non-perfect geographical population isolate of the Valserine valley [25], with a contribution of the relatively high level of geographical endogamy [74]. Finally, this variant spread within and outside the Rhône-Alpes region [25]. The mutation was also reported from clinical centers of Europe and North America (it might be identical with the original French cluster) [51], and also from Utah, US, in a family with ancestry to Ain, France [54]. Up to the present day, all families with c.1112_1113dupG variant can be traced back to the Rhône-Alpes region, confirming its founder effect.

The *ENG* c.67+1G>A pathogenic splice-site variant was detected in 7/10 unrelated families in the Curacao and Bonaire islands (population of 116,000 and 11,800 in 1998, respectively) of the Netherlands Antilles. The seven kindreds consisted of 58 affected individuals and 47 participated in the study of Gallione et al. [23]. Each proband had a shared core haplotype. At the time of the study, 102 HHT patients from 23 kindreds were living in Curacao and Bonaire, corresponding to a very high point-prevalence of 1:1331. In addition, this was an obvious underestimate, as only individuals above 12 years were assessed and only 70% of all known family members participated in the stratified population screening in the Afro-Caribbean population of the Netherlands Antilles [75]. The Dutch gained control over the temporarily nearly uninhabited islands in the middle of the 16th century and Curacao soon became the center of the Caribbean slave trade. The mutation could have been either of Antillean or African origin, although HHT is very rare in Sub-Saharan Africa [75,76]. The island as a past geographical population isolate and the relatively young age of the population are obvious. The variant was later also detected in the Netherlands in a family of Antillean origin [52].

The *ENG* c.360C>A pathogenic nonsense variant with a shared core haplotype was initially detected in 7/14 probands (50%), and furthermore, in 36/56 HHT patients (64.3%) with identified mutations from the island of Funen (Fyn), Denmark with a population of 470,000 in 1999 [44,66]. Mutation is estimated to have occurred 13 or 14 generations (approximately 340 years) before, either as a new variant or by immigration. Ten years later, in a Danish national HHT mutation study, 13 unrelated families were reported with this variant, that therefore, accounts for 13.68% (13/95) of all Danish kindreds with identified mutations. Otherwise, HHT point-prevalence was not extremely high in Funen (1:6410), as assessed by proband recruitment from hospital discharge records and subsequent family screening [21].

3.3. Potentially Grade IV Founder Variants

Five families and 38 affected individuals with the *ACVRL1* c.998G>T pathogenic missense variant were reported from Utah, US [50]. Genealogy revealed a common ancestor born in the early 1800s and his over 3000 at-risk living descendants. The local prevalence is unknown. This variant was detected in an additional American HHT family with four clinically affected individuals [43,51]. This family is geographically linked to the large Utah kindred, suggesting their common ancestry. A past geographical (varied landscape) or a cultural (relative young population by Mormon settlements in the mid-19th century) isolation might have occurred in Utah, but these are not referred by the authors.

Five families with 20 patients from two locations of Nordland, Norway, share the *ACVRL1* c.1450C>T pathogenic missense variant [48]. We have no information about the HHT prevalence in Nordland.

The *ENG* c.289-294delCACAAC indel variant was detected in 10 families with 40 affected individuals, residing in Bergamo County, Italy [29]. The authors emphasize that other HHT families with different mutations are also found in the population of 1,021,700 in 2007. Although very presumable, we cannot classify it straightaway as a grade IV variant in the lack local HHT prevalence data at that time. A past geographical isolation offered by the Alps in the northern part of the area is likely.

The *ENG* c.828_829insA variant was detected in six individuals of two large families with probands living in County A (population of 170,000 in 2002), Akita Prefecture, Japan [70]. A total of 15 patients in the two families were alive at the completion of the study. On the other hand, 23 known HHT patients were living in County A at that time, giving an approximate point-prevalence of 1:8000. We have no information about the number patients from the two concerned kindreds living in the study area. The study population is otherwise a past geographical isolate with founder effects of various genetic diseases like cholesteryl ester transfer protein (CETP) deficiency [77].

3.4. Tracing the Founder Event

Besides the above *ACVRL1* c.998G>T and c.1112_1113dupG variants, identical mutations with shared core haplotypes are sporadically observed in distinct populations. One of the two haplotypes of the *ACVRL1* c.200G>A (p.Arg67Gln) and one of the three haplotypes of the c.1120C>T (p.Arg374Trp) variants and the c.430C>T (p.Arg144*) variant are shared by French and Italian patients, and in the case of the latter two, the *DS12S1677* and *D12S296* marker alleles in the partially shared core haplotype are absent in the French control population. Thus, the common origin of these variants by Italian immigration to France, is likely [25].

The *ACVRL1* c.1121G>A (p.Arg374Gln) was initially described by Abdalla et al. [43], and later the variant was reported in three unrelated families in the US and France each, with ancestry from Deux-Sevres, France, in both cases. The French authors detected a common core haplotype. Based on the shared authorship of these publications, it is conceivable that these families are identical [25,51].

The *ACVRL1* c.1232G>A (p.Arg411Gln) variant is detected in two distantly related North American families with German and French origins, respectively [51]. Indeed, this variant was later reported from France and Germany [24,25,41]. On the other hand, it is present in several other unrelated populations, confirming a mutation hot-spot [38,39,60,62].

Two Antillean kindreds (four affected individuals) and a Dutch kindred (seven affected individuals) shared the *ENG* c.1238G>T missense mutation with a common core haplotype [23,78]. The Dutch family originates from Zeeland, the westernmost province of the Netherlands with extensive trading with the West Indies in the colonial times. The authors argue a potential European origin of this Antillean HHT mutation. The variant is reported from the Netherlands in another study of Letteboer et al. [52]. The European origin is further confirmed by the aforementioned fact that HHT is extremely rare in Sub-Saharan Africa [76].

3.5. Mutation Age

In order to estimate the age of the different founder events, likelihood-based methods were developed. Estimation is based on the size of the shared core haplotype flanking the mutation in the affected individuals, considering allele frequencies of the markers in the study population, likely recombination positions and mutation rates [25,44]. The mutation age is given with a confidence interval; the latter is highly influenced by the number of probands [25]. Two of the five founder variants with age estimates in the study of Lesca et al. showed regional clustering. One haplotype of the *ACVRL1* c.1121G>A (4 generations) in Deux-Sevres County was the youngest of all, while in the case of the c.1112_1113dupG (13 generations) variant in Jura and Ain Counties, the past partial geographical isolation could account for the still-existent clustering [25]. This might explain the dominance of the *ENG* c.360C>A variant with the same age in the island of Funen, Denmark, too [44]. In the

3.6. The Contribution of Genealogy

The main sources of genealogical tree reconstruction are parish registers (birth/christening, marriage and burial/death) and civil records from the late 17th century [74]. By means of genealogy, Letteboer at al found the common ancestor in three of the eight families with the *ENG* c.781T>C variant in 1765, in five of the seven families with the *ACVRL1* c.1042delG variant in 1722 and in all five families with the *ENG* c.1311G>A variant in 1745, respectively [52]. The six families with the *ACVRL1* c.625+1G>C variant and its shared core haplotype could be traced back to a single founder in 1779 [46]. A co-existence of several favorable circumstances supported our effort. First, original parish registers were not destroyed by wars or natural forces. Second, in Hungary surnames are identical with family names (and not patronymics, for instance). Our HHT kindreds beared infrequent family names. Third, non-paternity probably did not occur in our series. Fourth, pedigree charts of the six families met at a time following the introduction of parish registers. Though prescribed by Pope Pius IV in the Council of Trent in 1563 [79], Catholic church registers were introduced at the beginning of the 18th century in Hungary. We emphasize that the identified common ancestor of the concerned families is not inevitably identical with the founder of the mutation in the population. Further families with this variant sharing a less correspondent haplotype might be identified whenever in the future, suggesting a more remote common ancestor [46].

However, many genealogical links might be found between affected families, resulting in a non-absolute genealogical convergence of the ancestors [22,74]. Tracing the pedigrees of 49 families living or originating in five contiguous villages of the Valserine Valley, 47,000 parish and 6000 civil records covering three centuries were reviewed, resulting in a dense network of common ancestors. Finally, 929 individuals in the mid-17th century were found at the top of the genealogical trees. The possible founder(s) should be among them [22]. The genetic tests performed more than a decade later revealed several causative variants in this area, in addition to the French founder one. An additional example for the multiple common ancestries of two Hungarian HHT families with the *ENG* c.817-2A>C mutation is shown in Supplementary Materials Figure S2 [42]. In conclusion, in the molecular genetic era, genealogy plays an auxiliary role in the identification of founder effects. We propose the thorough medical pedigree construction up to the farthest ancestors with HHT symptoms by alive kindred individuals' hearsay and keeping of registers with HHT family names.

3.7. How Can an Autosomal Dominant Disease Like HHT Result in a Founder Effect?

The fate of a potential founder allele is a combination of genetic drift and selection. There is evidence for some of the frequent founder mutations in recessive diseases to confer a selective advantage to heterozygotes (e.g., the G6PD^{Med} mutation resulting in malaria resistance) [4]. Selection might have a neutral or a slight negative impact on the founder effects in HHT. In a population genetic study performed by Kjeldsen et al. in Funen, Denmark, more than two decades ago, HHT was found to associate with an excess mortality, particularly in patients below the age of 60 years at inclusion. In this latter group, the cumulative mortality rate was twofold of the age- and gender-matched controls, and this rise was exclusively attributable to HHT complications as bleeding and pulmonary arteriovenous malformations (PAVMs) [21]. Major complications from undiagnosed PAVMs like paradoxical emboli (leading to ischemic stroke or brain abscess) or hemothorax significantly reduce the quality of life and life expectancy of HHT patients [80,81]. On the other hand, penetrance is age-related, and these complications have no significant effect on reproductive fitness, permitting HHT to result in a founder effect. This might be particularly the case in HHT2 with occasionally later onset of symptoms [46,50,82] and definitely lower prevalence of potentially fatal PAVMs, compared to HHT1 [45,54,67]. Indeed, two-thirds of the founder mutations affect the *ACVRL1* gene.

4. The Significance of Founder Effects

The bigger the cluster of HHT families and patients with a founder variant, the more remarkable is its influence to the HHT1/HHT2 ratio in a certain administrative area [23,24,46–48,66] or even nationwide, slightly affecting the HHT phenotype [29,48,67]. On the other hand, the phenotypes of HHT1 and HHT2 are overlapping, and according to the International HHT Guidelines released in 2011 and its 2020 revision [83,84], neither the diagnostic nor the management algorithms differ in HHT1 and HHT2.

Similar to the second-hit hypothesis of familiar cancers, an environmental (inflammation, hypoxia, sunlight, trauma) or a genetic (a somatic mutation in the wild-type allele of HHT genes or a germline variant in modifiers) second-hit added to the germline HHT mutation [85], might explain the focal appearance of vascular lesions, the age-related penetrance and the considerable intrafamilial variance in HHT phenotype [23,50,52,66]. Founding kindreds, especially the larger ones with more uniform core haplotypes and living in uniform environmental conditions, might be theoretical targets for these genetic second-hit studies.

When one or a few founder variants account for the majority of all pathogenic variants found in a population, testing for the founder(s) may be performed first [10]. Considering the International HHT Guidelines [84], this screening might refer exclusively to the pathogenic variants and each of them appearing in the study area must be tested simultaneously. However, relying on merely to the founder screening carries some risks. Non-founder variants also presenting in the area [25,66,70] might be overlooked. Furthermore, in the nationwide study of Heimdal et al. [48], a family with the pathogenic missense *ACVRL* c.1450C>T founder and a likely pathogenic *ACVRL1* c.11delG variant in cis were reported. This might be also overlooked by screening for founder mutations only. With the availability of Next-Generation Sequencing, many labs would find it cost and time efficient to sequence the entire gene(s). In our practice, we screen for the known local founder mutations in new families with HHT phenotype as first-line test and accept them as the causative variants in the case of co-segregation. If no founder mutation is found in the patient, second-line genetic investigations including all HHT causative genes are performed.

5. Limitations

The references in the HHT Mutation Database are not necessarily up-to-date, as a number of recently detected HHT variants are not submitted. A part of these variants could have been missed by the subsequent PubMed and Scopus search, especially the ones that were not considered as founder by the authors.

With very few exceptions, all the listed data (Table 2) originate from European or North American subpopulations, resulting in a publication bias.

The ambiguous definitions of "apparently unrelated families", "shared area of ancestry or residence", "shared core haplotype", "genealogical evidence of common ancestry" and the arbitrary grading system could either under- or overestimate certain variants as founders. The definition of the "founder effect" itself and, furthermore, the minimal population size for the investigation of founder effects are equivocal in the literature. Theoretically a single large resident family with an exactly kept genealogical tree might result in a founder effect in a small population, especially if it is thoroughly screened, like the kindred with the *ACVRL1* c.1120C>T in the paper of Kjeldsen et al. [55]. Neither the affected kindred nor the study population sizes could be retrieved from the majority of the revised papers.

Interestingly, the *ENG* c.277C>T (p.Arg93*) was detected in 12 patients from five unrelated families from various locations in Southeastern Norway [48]. This would have been a grade III founder effect by our grading system, but subsequent haplotype analysis showed different haplotypes and the authors reported it as a hot-spot. Thus, we reclassified it as a repetitive mutation (grade I). Though the c.277C>T variant is reported by a number of authors, confirming the hot-spot [29,44,49,52,59,86], its clustering with distinct haplotypes within a geographical area is surprising. This could have occurred in any of the cases categorized as an even grade III variant merely upon the shared area of ancestry or residence.

6. Conclusions

Although HHT is inherited in an autosomal dominant trait and present population isolates with HHT are not known, some causative *ACVRL1* and *ENG* variants are reported with variable evidences for founder effects. This might be attributable to the age-related penetrance, without a significant effect on reproductive fitness. Being aware of local founder variants might simplify HHT gene testing in specific populations, with some potential pitfalls. Large founding kindreds might be potential targets for genetic second-hit studies.

Supplementary Materials: The following are available online at https://www.mdpi.com/article/10.3390/jcm10081682/s1. Figure S1: Haplotype analysis of patients and unaffected individuals in seven families with the *ACVRL1* c.625+1G>C mutation [46]. Figure S2: Common ancestry of two families exhibiting the ENG c.817-2A>C mutation [42]. Table S1: Publications corresponding to any of the terms *"founder"* and *"founding"* and the etymon *"ancest"*. Table S2: Reassessment of pathogenicity of variants reported as "pending" in the *ENG* and *ACVRL1* Databases [26,27].

Author Contributions: Conceptualization, T.M. and Z.B.; literature search, T.M. and R.G.; software, G.B.; reconstruction of genealogical trees by parish registers, P.B.; writing—original draft preparation, T.M.; writing—review and editing, R.G. and P.B.; supervision, Z.B. All authors have read and agreed to the published version of the manuscript.

Funding: This research was funded by the European Union under European Regional Development Fund, grant number GINOP-2.3.2-15-2016-00039 and by the National Research, Development and Innovation Office, Hungarian Ministry of Innovation and Technology, grant number OTKA K116228. The APC was funded by University of Debrecen.

Institutional Review Board Statement: Not applicable.

Informed Consent Statement: Not applicable.

Conflicts of Interest: The authors declare no conflict of interest.

References

1. Slatkin, M. A Population-Genetic Test of Founder Effects and Implications for Ashkenazi Jewish Diseases. *Am. J. Hum. Genet.* **2004**, *75*, 282–293. [CrossRef]
2. Arcos-Burgos, M.; Muenke, M. Genetics of population isolates. *Clin. Genet.* **2002**, *61*, 233–247. [CrossRef]
3. Payne, M.; Rupar, C.A.; Siu, G.M.; Siu, V.M. Amish, Mennonite, and Hutterite Genetic Disorder Database. *Paediatr. Child Health* **2011**, *16*, e23–e24. [CrossRef]
4. Ostrer, H.; Skorecki, K. The population genetics of the Jewish people. *Hum. Genet.* **2012**, *132*, 119–127. [CrossRef]
5. Francomano, C.A.; McKusick, V.A.; Biesecker, L.G. Medical genetic studies in the Amish: Historical perspective. *Am. J. Med. Genet.* **2003**, *121C*, 1–4. [CrossRef]
6. Charrow, J. Ashkenazi Jewish genetic disorders. *Fam. Cancer* **2004**, *3*, 201–206. [CrossRef]
7. Orton, N.C.; Innes, A.M.; Chudley, A.E.; Bech-Hansen, N.T. Unique disease heritage of the Dutch-German Mennonite population. *Am. J. Med. Genet.* **2008**, *146A*, 1072–1087. [CrossRef]
8. Pisano, M.; Cossu, A.; Persico, I.; Palmieri, G.; Angius, A.; Casu, G.; Palomba, G.; Sarobba, M.G.; Ossu Rocca, P.C.; Dedola, M.F.; et al. Identification of a founder BRCA2 mutation in Sardinia. *Br. J. Cancer* **2000**, *82*, 553–559. [CrossRef]
9. Dagan, E.; Gershoni-Baruch, R.; Kurolap, A.; Fried, G. Early onset breast cancer in Ashkenazi women carriers of founder BRCA1/2 mutations: Beyond 10 years of follow-up. *Eur. J. Cancer Care* **2016**, *26*, e12594. [CrossRef]
10. Wallace, S.E.; Bean, L.J.H. *Resources for Genetics Professionals—Genetic Disorders Associated with Founder Variants Common in the Druze Population*; Adam, M.P., Ardinger, H.H., Pagon, R.A., Eds.; GeneReviews®: Seattle, WA, USA, 2019. Available online: https://www.ncbi.nlm.nih.gov/books/NBK549466/ (accessed on 25 February 2021).
11. Borst, A.J.; Nakano, T.A.; Blei, F.; Adams, D.M.; Duis, J. A Primer on a Comprehensive Genetic Approach to Vascular Anomalies. *Front. Pediatr.* **2020**, *8*. [CrossRef]

12. About Rare Diseases. Available online: https://www.12/consor/cgi-bin/Education_AboutRareDiseases.php?lng=EN (accessed on 24 February 2021).
13. McDonald, J.; Wooderchak-Donahue, W.; Van Sant Webb, C.; Whitehead, K.; Stevenson, D.A.; Bayrak-Toydemir, P. Hereditary hemorrhagic telangiectasia: Genetics and molecular diagnostics in a new era. *Front. Genet.* **2015**, *6*, 1–8. [CrossRef]
14. Sharathkumar, A.A.; Shapiro, A. Hereditary haemorrhagic telangiectasia. *Haemophilia* **2008**, *14*, 1269–1280. [CrossRef] [PubMed]
15. McAllister, K.A.; Grogg, K.M.; Johnson, D.W.; Gallione, C.J.; Baldwin, M.A.; Jackson, C.E.; Helmbold, E.A.; Markel, D.S.; McKinnon, W.C.; Murrell, J. Endoglin, a TGF-beta binding protein of endothelial cells, is the gene for hereditary haemorrhagic telangiectasia type 1. *Nat. Genet.* **1994**, *8*, 345–351. [CrossRef]
16. Johnson, D.W.; Berg, L.N.; Baldwin, M.A.; Gallione, C.J.; Marondel, I.; Yoon, S.J.; Stenzel, T.T.; Speer, M.; Pericak-Vance, M.A.; Diamond, A.; et al. Mutations in the activin receptor-like kinase 1 gene in hereditary haemorrhagic telangiectasia type 2. *Nat. Genet.* **1996**, *13*, 189–195. [CrossRef] [PubMed]
17. Plauchu, H.; De Chadarévian, J.-P.; Bideau, A.; Robert, J.-M. Age-related clinical profile of hereditary hemorrhagic telangiectasia in an epidemiologically recruited population. *Am. J. Med. Genet.* **1989**, *32*, 291–297. [CrossRef]
18. Jessurun, G.A.; Nossent, J.C. Cerebrovascular accidents at a young age in Rendu-Osler-Weber disease; a survey in the Netherlands Antilles. *Ned. Tijdschr. Geneeskd.* **1992**, *136*, 428–431. [PubMed]
19. Porteous, M.E.; Burn, J.; Proctor, S.J. Hereditary haemorrhagic telangiectasia: A clinical analysis. *J. Med. Genet.* **1992**, *29*, 527–530. [CrossRef] [PubMed]
20. Guttmacher, A.E.; McKinnon, W.C.; Upton, M.D. Hereditary haemorrhagic telangiectasia: A disorder in search of the genetics community. *Am. J. Med. Genet.* **1994**, *52*, 252–253. [CrossRef] [PubMed]
21. Kjeldsen, A.D.; Vase, P.; Green, A. Hereditary haemorrhagic telangiectasia: A population-based study of prevalence and mortality in Danish patients. *J. Intern. Med.* **1999**, *245*, 31–39. [CrossRef]
22. Bideau, A.; Brunet, G.; Heyer, E.; Plauchu, H.; Robert, J.-M. An abnormal concentration of cases of Rendu-Osler disease in the Valserine valley of the French Jura: A genealogical and demographic study. *Ann. Hum. Biol.* **1992**, *19*, 233–247. [CrossRef] [PubMed]
23. Gallione, C.J.; Scheessele, E.A.; Reinhardt, D.; Duits, A.J.; Berg, J.N.; Westermann, C.J.J.; Marchuk, D.A. Two common endoglin mutations in families with hereditary hemorrhagic telangiectasia in the Netherlands Antilles: Evidence for a founder effect. *Hum. Genet.* **2000**, *107*, 40–44. [CrossRef] [PubMed]
24. Lesca, G.; Plauchu, H.; Coulet, F.; Lefebvre, S.; Plessis, G.; Odent, S.; Rivière, S.; Leheup, B.; Goizet, C.; Carette, M.-F.; et al. Molecular screening of ALK1/ACVRL1 and ENG genes in hereditary hemorrhagic telangiectasia in France. *Hum. Mutat.* **2004**, *23*, 289–299. [CrossRef] [PubMed]
25. Lesca, G.; Genin, E.; Blachier, C.; Olivieri, C.; Coulet, F.; Brunet, G.; Dupuis-Girod, S.; Buscarini, E.; Soubrier, F.; Calender, A.; et al. Hereditary hemorrhagic telangiectasia: Evidence for regional founder effects of ACVRL1 mutations in French and Italian patients. *Eur. J. Hum. Genet.* **2008**, *16*, 742–749. [CrossRef]
26. ENG Database. Available online: https://arup.utah.edu/database/ENG/ENG_display.php (accessed on 7 February 2021).
27. ACVRL1 Database. Available online: https://arup.utah.edu/database/ACVRL1/ACVRL1_display.php (accessed on 7 February 2021).
28. SMAD4 Dabase. Available online: https://arup.utah.edu/database/SMAD4/SMAD4_display.php (accessed on 7 February 2021).
29. Olivieri, C.; Pagella, F.; Semino, L.; Lanzarini, L.; Valacca, C.; Pilotto, A.; Corno, S.; Scappaticci, S.; Manfredi, G.; Buscarini, E.; et al. Analysis of ENG and ACVRL1 genes in 137 HHT Italian families identifies 76 different mutations (24 novel). Comparison with other European studies. *J. Hum. Genet.* **2007**, *52*, 820–829. [CrossRef]
30. Richards, S.; Aziz, N.; Bale, S.; Bick, D.; Das, S.; Gastier-Foster, J.; Grody, W.W.; Hegde, M.; Lyon, E.; Spector, E.; et al. Standards and guidelines for the interpretation of sequence variants: A joint consensus recommendation of the American College of Medical Genetics and Genomics and the Association for Molecular Pathology. *Genet. Med.* **2015**, *17*, 405–423. [CrossRef]
31. Giordano, P.; Nigro, A.; Lenato, G.M.; Guanti, G.; Suppressa, P.; Lastella, P.; De Mattia, D.; Sabba, C. Screening for children from families with Rendu-Osler-Weber disease: From geneticist to clinician. *J. Thromb. Haemost.* **2006**, *4*, 1237–1245. [CrossRef]
32. Ricard, N.; Bidart, M.; Mallet, C.; Lesca, G.; Giraud, S.; Prudent, R.; Feige, J.-J.; Bailly, S. Functional analysis of the BMP9 response of ALK1 mutants from HHT2 patients: A diagnostic tool for novel ACVRL1 mutations. *Blood* **2010**, *116*, 1604–1612. [CrossRef]
33. Olivieri, C.; Mira, E.; Delù, G.; Pagella, F.; Zambelli, A.; Malvezzi, L.; Buscarini, E.; Danesino, C. Identification of 13 new mutations in the ACVRL1 gene in a group of 52 unselected Italian patients affected by hereditary haemorrhagic telangiectasia. *J. Med. Genet.* **2002**, *39*, e39. [CrossRef]
34. Abdalla, S.A.; Cymerman, U.; Rushlow, D.; Chen, N.; Stoeber, G.P.; Lemire, E.G.; Letarte, M. Novel mutations and polymorphisms in genes causing hereditary hemorrhagic telangiectasia. *Hum. Mutat.* **2005**, *25*, 320–321. [CrossRef]
35. Kuehl, H.K.; Caselitz, M.; Hasenkamp, S.; Wagner, S.; El-Harith, H.A.; Manns, M.P.; Stuhrmann, M. Hepatic manifestation is associated with ALK1 in hereditary hemorrhagic telangiectasia: Identification of five novel ALK1 and one novel ENG mutations. *Hum. Mutat.* **2005**, *25*, 320. [CrossRef]
36. Ha, M.; Kim, Y.J.; Kwon, K.A.; Hahm, K.B.; Kim, M.J.; Kim, D.K.; Lee, Y.J.; Oh, S.P. Gastric angiodysplasia in a hereditary hemorrhagic telangiectasia type 2 patient. *World J. Gastroenterol.* **2012**, *18*, 1840–1844. [CrossRef] [PubMed]

37. Chen, Y.-J.; Yang, Q.-H.; Liu, D.; Liu, Q.-Q.; Eyries, M.; Wen, L.; Jiang, X.; Yuan, P.; Zhang, R.; Soubrier, F.; et al. Clinical and genetic characteristics of Chinese patients with hereditary haemorrhagic telangiectasia-associated pulmonary hypertension. *Eur. J. Clin. Investig.* **2013**, *43*, 1016–1024. [CrossRef]
38. Berg, J.N.; Gallione, C.J.; Stenzel, T.T.; Johnson, D.W.; Allen, W.P.; Schwartz, C.E.; Jackson, C.E.; Porteous, M.E.; Marchuk, D.A. The activin receptor-like kinase 1 gene: Genomic structure and mutations in hereditary hemorrhagic telangiectasia type 2. *Am. J. Hum. Genet.* **1997**, *61*, 60–67. [CrossRef]
39. Schulte, C.; Geisthoff, U.; Lux, A.; Kupka, S.; Zenner, H.P.; Blin, N.; Pfister, M. High frequency of ENG and ALK1/ACVRL1 mutations in German HHT patients. *Hum. Mutat.* **2005**, *25*, 595. [CrossRef] [PubMed]
40. Lenato, G.M.; Lastella, P.; Di Giacomo, M.C.; Resta, N.; Suppressa, P.; Pasculli, G.; Sabbà, C.; Guanti, G. DHPLC-based mutation analysis of ENG and ALK-1 genes in HHT Italian population. *Hum. Mutat.* **2006**, *27*, 213–214. [CrossRef]
41. Zhao, Y.; Zhang, Y.; Wang, X.; Zhang, L. Variant analysis in Chinese families with hereditary hemorrhagic telangiectasia. *Mol. Genet. Genom. Med.* **2019**, *7*, e893. [CrossRef]
42. Major, T.; Gindele, R.; Szabó, Z.; Jóni, N.; Kis, Z.; Bora, L.; Bárdossy, P.; Rácz, T.; Karosi, T.; Bereczky, Z. A heredíter haemorrhagiás teleangiectasia (Osler–Weber–Rendu-kór) genetikai diagnosztikája. *Orv. Hetil.* **2019**, *160*, 710–719. [CrossRef]
43. Abdalla, S.A.; Cymerman, U.; Johnson, R.M.; Deber, C.M.; Letarte, M. Disease-associated mutations in conserved residues of ALK-1 kinase domain. *Eur. J. Hum. Genet.* **2003**, *11*, 279–287. [CrossRef]
44. Brusgaard, K.; Kjeldsen, A.; Poulsen, L.; Moss, H.; Vase, P.; Rasmussen, K.; Kruse, T.A.; Hørder, M. Mutations in endoglin and in activin receptor-like kinase 1 among Danish patients with hereditary haemorrhagic telangiectasia. *Clin. Genet.* **2004**, *66*, 556–561. [CrossRef] [PubMed]
45. Komiyama, M.; Ishiguro, T.; Yamada, O.; Morisaki, H.; Morisaki, T. Hereditary hemorrhagic telangiectasia in Japanese patients. *J. Hum. Genet.* **2014**, *59*, 37–41. [CrossRef]
46. Major, T.; Gindele, R.; Szabó, Z.; Alef, T.; Thiele, B.; Bora, L.; Kis, Z.; Bárdossy, P.; Rácz, T.; Havacs, I.; et al. Evidence for the founder effect of a novel ACVRL1 splice-site mutation in Hungarian hereditary hemorrhagic telangiectasia families. *Clin. Genet.* **2016**, *90*, 466–467. [CrossRef]
47. Major, T.; Gindele, R.; Szabó, Z.; Kis, Z.; Bora, L.; Jóni, N.; Bárdossy, P.; Rácz, T.; Bereczky, Z. The Stratified Population Screening of Hereditary Hemorrhagic Telangiectasia. *Pathol. Oncol. Res.* **2020**, *26*, 2783–2788. [CrossRef]
48. Heimdal, K.; Dalhus, B.; Rødningen, O.K.; Kroken, M.; Eiklid, K.; Dheyauldeen, S.; Røysland, T.; Andersen, R.; Kulseth, M.A. Mutation analysis in Norwegian families with hereditary hemorrhagic telangiectasia: Founder mutations in ACVRL1. *Clin. Genet.* **2015**, *89*, 182–186. [CrossRef]
49. Bossler, A.D.; Richards, J.; George, C.; Godmilow, L.; Ganguly, A. Novel mutations in ENG and ACVRL1 identified in a series of 200 individuals undergoing clinical genetic testing for hereditary hemorrhagic telangiectasia (HHT): Correlation of genotype with phenotype. *Hum. Mutat.* **2006**, *27*, 667–675. [CrossRef] [PubMed]
50. McDonald, J.E.; Miller, F.J.; Hallam, S.E.; Nelson, L.; Marchuk, D.A.; Ward, K.J. Clinical manifestations in a large hereditary hemorrhagic telangiectasia (HHT) type 2 kindred. *Am. J. Med. Genet.* **2000**, *93*, 320–327. [CrossRef]
51. Abdalla, S.A.; Geisthoff, U.W.; Bonneau, D.; Plauchu, H.; McDonald, J.; Kennedy, S.; Faughnan, M.E.; Letarte, M. Visceral manifestations in hereditary haemorrhagictelangiectasia type 2. *J. Med. Genet.* **2003**, *40*, 494–502. [CrossRef]
52. Letteboer, T.G.W.; Zewald, R.A.; Kamping, E.J.; de Haas, G.; Mager, J.J.; Snijder, R.J.; Lindhout, D.; Hennekam, F.A.M.; Westermann, C.J.J.; Ploos van Amstel, J.K. Hereditary hemorrhagic telangiectasia: ENG and ALK-1 mutations in Dutch patients. *Hum. Genet.* **2004**, *116*, 8–16. [CrossRef]
53. Smoot, L.B.; Obler, D.; McElhinney, D.B.; Boardman, K.; Wu, B.-L.; Lip, V.; Mullen, M.P. Clinical features of pulmonary arterial hypertension in young people with an ALK1 mutation and hereditary haemorrhagic telangiectasia. *Arch. Dis. Child.* **2009**, *94*, 506–511. [CrossRef]
54. Bayrak-Toydemir, P.; McDonald, J.; Markewitz, B.; Lewin, S.; Miller, F.; Chou, L.; Gedge, F.; Tang, W.; Coon, H.; Mao, R. Genotype-phenotype correlation in hereditary hemorrhagic telangiectasia: Mutations and manifestations. *Am. J. Med. Genet.* **2006**, *140*, 463–470. [CrossRef]
55. Kjeldsen, A.D.; Brusgaard, K.; Poulsen, L.; Kruse, T.; Rasmussen, K.; Green, A.; Vase, P. Mutations in theALK-1 gene and the phenotype of hereditary hemorrhagic telangiectasia in two large Danish families. *Am. J. Med. Genet.* **2001**, *98*, 298–302. [CrossRef]
56. Harrison, R.E.; Flanagan, J.A.; Sankelo, M.; Abdalla, S.A.; Rowell, J.; Machado, R.D.; Elliott, C.G.; Robbins, I.M.; Olschewski, H.; McLaughlin, V.; et al. Molecular and functional analysis identifies ALK-1 as the predominant cause of pulmonary hypertension related to hereditary haemorrhagic telangiectasia. *J. Med. Genet.* **2003**, *40*, 865–871. [CrossRef]
57. Sanz-Rodriguez, F.; Fernandez-L, A.; Zarrabeitia, R.; Perez-Molino, A.; Ramírez, J.R.; Coto, E.; Bernabeu, C.; Botella, L.M. Mutation analysis in Spanish patients with hereditary hemorrhagic telangiectasia: Deficient endoglin up-regulation in activated monocytes. *Clin. Chem.* **2004**, *50*, 2003–2011. [CrossRef]
58. Wehner, L.-E.; Folz, B.; Argyriou, L.; Twelkemeyer, S.; Teske, U.; Geisthoff, U.; Wernerb, J.A.; Engel, W.; Nayernia, K. Mutation analysis in hereditary haemorrhagic telangiectasia in Germany reveals 11 novel ENG and 12 novel ACVRL1/ALK1 mutations. *Clin. Genet.* **2006**, *69*, 239–245. [CrossRef]
59. Gedge, F.; McDonald, J.; Phansalkar, A.; Chou, L.S.; Calderon, F.; Mao, R.; Lyon, E.; Bayrak-Toydemir, P. Clinical and analytical sensitivities in hereditary hemorrhagic telangiectasia testing and a report of de novo mutations. *J. Mol. Diagn.* **2007**, *9*, 258–265. [CrossRef]

60. Fontalba, A.; Fernandez-L, A.; García-Alegría, E.; Albiñana, V.; Garrido-Martin, E.M.; Blanco, F.J.; Zarrabeitia, R.; Perez-Molino, A.; Bernabeu-Herrero, M.E.; Ojeda, M.-L.; et al. Mutation study of Spanish patients with Hereditary Hemorrhagic Telangiectasia. *BMC Med. Genet.* **2008**, *9*. [CrossRef]
61. Trembath, R.C.; Thomson, J.R.; Machado, R.D.; Morgan, N.V.; Atkinson, C.; Winship, I.; Simonneau, G.; Galie, N.; Loyd, J.E.; Humbert, M.; et al. Clinical and molecular genetic features of pulmonary hypertension in patients with hereditary hemorrhagic telangiectasia. *N. Engl. J. Med.* **2001**, *345*, 325–334. [CrossRef]
62. Lin, W.D.; Wu, J.Y.; Hsu, H.B.; Tsai, F.J.; Lee, C.C.; Tsai, C.H. Mutation analysis of a family with hereditary hemorrhagic telangiectasia associated with hepatic arteriovenous malformation. *J. Formos. Med. Assoc.* **2001**, *100*, 817–819.
63. Abdalla, S.A.; Gallione, C.J.; Barst, R.J.; Horn, E.M.; Knowles, J.A.; Marchuk, D.A.; Letarte, M.; Morse, J.H. Primary pulmonary hypertension in families with hereditary haemorrhagic telangiectasia. *Eur. Respir. J.* **2004**, *23*, 373–377. [CrossRef]
64. Yan, Z.M.; Fan, Z.P.; Du, J.; Hua, H.; Xu, Y.Y.; Wang, S.L. A novel mutation in ALK-1 causes hereditary hemorrhagic telangiectasia type 2. *J. Dent. Res.* **2006**, *85*, 705–710. [CrossRef]
65. Lesca, G.; Burnichon, N.; Raux, G.; Tosi, M.; Pinson, S.; Marion, M.J.; Babin, E.; Gilbert-Dussardier, B.; Rivière, S.; Goizet, C.; et al. French Rendu-Osler Network. Distribution of ENG and ACVRL1 (ALK1) mutations in French HHT patients. *Hum. Mutat.* **2006**, *27*, 598. [CrossRef]
66. Kjeldsen, A.D.; Moller, T.R.; Brusgaard, K.; Vase, P.; Andersen, P.E. Clinical symptoms according to genotype amongst patients with hereditary haemorrhagic telangiectasia. *J. Intern. Med.* **2005**, *258*, 349–355. [CrossRef] [PubMed]
67. Tørring, P.M.; Brusgaard, K.; Ousager, L.B.; Andersen, P.E.; Kjeldsen, A.D. National mutation study among Danish patients with hereditary haemorrhagic telangiectasia. *Clin. Genet.* **2013**, *86*, 123–133. [CrossRef]
68. Pece, N.; Vera, S.; Cymerman, U.; White, R.I., Jr.; Wrana, J.L.; Letarte, M. Mutant endoglin in hereditary hemorrhagic telangiectasia type 1 is transiently expressed intracellularly and is not a dominant negative. *J. Clin. Investig.* **1997**, *100*, 2568–2579. [CrossRef] [PubMed]
69. Kim, M.J.; Kim, S.T.; Lee, H.D.; Lee, K.Y.; Seo, J.; Lee, J.B.; Lee, Y.J.; Oh, S.P. Clinical and genetic analyses of three Korean families with hereditary hemorrhagic telangiectasia. *BMC Med. Genet.* **2011**, *12*, 130. [CrossRef] [PubMed]
70. Dakeishi, M.; Shioya, T.; Wada, Y.; Shindo, T.; Otaka, K.; Manabe, M.; Nozaki, J.; Inoue, S.; Koizumi, A. Genetic epidemiology of hereditary hemorrhagic telangiectasia in a local community in the northern part of Japan. *Hum. Mutat.* **2002**, *19*, 140–148. [CrossRef] [PubMed]
71. Shovlin, C.L.; Hughes, J.M.B.; Scott, J.; Seidman, C.E.; Seidman, J.G. Characterization of Endoglin and Identification of Novel Mutations in Hereditary Hemorrhagic Telangiectasia. *Am. J. Hum. Genet.* **1997**, *61*, 68–79. [CrossRef]
72. Wooderchak-Donahue, W.L.; McDonald, J.; O'Fallon, B.; Upton, P.D.; Li, W.; Roman, B.L.; Young, S.; Plant, P.; Fulop, G.T.; Langa, C.; et al. BMP9 Mutations Cause a Vascular-Anomaly Syndrome with Phenotypic Overlap with Hereditary Hemorrhagic Telangiectasia. *Am. J. Hum. Genet.* **2013**, *93*, 530–537. [CrossRef]
73. Hernandez, F.; Huether, R.; Carter, L.; Johnston, T.; Thompson, J.; Gossage, J.R.; Chao, E.; Elliott, A.M. Mutations in RASA1 and GDF2 identified in patients with clinical features of hereditary hemorrhagic telangiectasia. *Hum. Genome Var.* **2015**, *2*, 15040. [CrossRef]
74. Brunet, G.; Lesca, G.; Génin, E.; Dupuis-Girod, S.; Bideau, A.; Plauchu, H. Thirty Years of Research into Rendu-Osler-Weber Disease in France: Historical Demography, Population Genetics and Molecular Biology. *Population* **2009**, 273–291. [CrossRef]
75. Westermann, C.J.J.; Rosina, A.F.; de Vries, v.; de Coteau, P.A. The prevalence and manifestations of hereditary hemorrhagic telangiectasia in the Afro-Caribbean population of the Netherlands Antilles: A family screening. *Am. J. Med. Genet.* **2003**, *116*, 324–328. [CrossRef]
76. Canzonieri, C.; Ornati, F.; Matti, E.; Chu, F.; Manfredi, G.; Olivieri, C.; Buscarini, E.; Pagella, F. Hereditary haemorrhagic telangiectasia in North African and sub-Saharan patients. *S. Afr. Med. J.* **2014**, *104*, 256–257. [CrossRef] [PubMed]
77. Hirano, K.; Yamashita, S.; Nakajima, N.; Arai, T.; Maruyama, T.; Yoshida, Y.; Ishigami, M.; Sakai, N.; Kameda-Takemura, K.; Matsuzawa, Y. Genetic cholesteryl ester transfer protein deficiency is extremely frequent in the Omagari area of Japan. Marked hyperalphalipoproteinemia caused by CETP gene mutation is not associated with longevity. *Arterioscler. Thromb. Vasc. Biol.* **1997**, *17*, 1053–1059. [CrossRef]
78. Heutink, P.; Haitjema, T.; Breedveld, G.J.; Janssen, B.; Sandkuijl, L.A.; Bontekoe, C.J.; Westerman, C.J.; Oostra, B.A. Linkage of hereditary haemorrhagic telangiectasia to chromosome 9q34 and evidence for locus heterogeneity. *J. Med. Genet.* **1994**, *31*, 933–936. [CrossRef] [PubMed]
79. Laplante, B. From France to the Church: The Generalization of Parish Registers in the Catholic Countries. *J. Fam. Hist.* **2018**, *44*, 24–51. [CrossRef]
80. Donaldson, J.W.; McKeever, T.M.; Hall, I.P.; Hubbard, R.B.; Fogarty, A.W. Complications and mortality in hereditary hemorrhagic telangiectasia: A population-based study. *Neurology* **2015**, *84*, 1886–1893. [CrossRef]
81. de Gussem, E.M.; Edwards, C.P.; Hosman, A.E.; Westermann, C.J.; Snijder, R.J.; Faughnan, M.E.; Mager, J.J. Life expectancy of parents with Hereditary Haemorrhagic Telangiectasia. *Orphanet J. Rare Dis.* **2016**, *22*, 11–46. [CrossRef]
82. Brakensiek, K.; Frye-Boukhriss, H.; Mälzer, M.; Abramowicz, M.; Bahr, M.J.; von Beckerath, N.; Bergmann, C.; Caselitz, M.; Holinski-Feder, E.; Muschke, P.; et al. Detection of a significant association between mutations in the ACVRL1 gene and hepatic involvement in German patients with hereditary haemorrhagic telangiectasia. *Clin. Genet.* **2008**, *74*, 171–777. [CrossRef]

83. Faughnan, M.E.; Palda, V.A.; Garcia-Tsao, G.; Geisthoff, U.W.; McDonald, J.; Proctor, D.D.; Spears, J.; Brown, D.H.; Buscarini, E.; Chesnutt, M.S.; et al. HHT Foundation International—Guidelines Working Group. International guidelines for the diagnosis and management of hereditary haemorrhagic telangiectasia. *J. Med. Genet.* **2011**, *48*, 73–87. [CrossRef]
84. Faughnan, M.E.; Mager, J.J.; Hetts, S.W.; Palda, V.A.; Lang-Robertson, K.; Buscarini, E.; Deslandres, E.; Kasthuri, R.S.; Lausman, A.; Poetker, D.; et al. Second International Guidelines for the Diagnosis and Management of Hereditary Hemorrhagic Telangiectasia. *Ann. Intern. Med.* **2020**, *15*, 989–1001. [CrossRef]
85. Bernabeu, C.; Bayrak-Toydemir, P.; McDonald, J.; Letarte, M. Potential Second-Hits in Hereditary Hemorrhagic Telangiectasia. *J. Clin. Med.* **2020**, *9*, 3571. [CrossRef]
86. Nishida, T.; Faughnan, M.E.; Krings, T.; Chakinala, M.; Gossage, J.R.; Young, W.L.; Kim, H.; Pourmohamad, T.; Henderson, K.J.; Schrum, S.D.; et al. Brain arteriovenous malformations associated with hereditary hemorrhagic telangiectasia: Gene-phenotype correlations. *Am. J. Med. Genet.* **2012**, *158A*, 2829–2834. [CrossRef] [PubMed]

MDPI
St. Alban-Anlage 66
4052 Basel
Switzerland
www.mdpi.com

Journal of Clinical Medicine Editorial Office
E-mail: jcm@mdpi.com
www.mdpi.com/journal/jcm

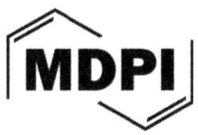

Disclaimer/Publisher's Note: The statements, opinions and data contained in all publications are solely those of the individual author(s) and contributor(s) and not of MDPI and/or the editor(s). MDPI and/or the editor(s) disclaim responsibility for any injury to people or property resulting from any ideas, methods, instructions or products referred to in the content.

www.ingramcontent.com/pod-product-compliance
Lightning Source LLC
LaVergne TN
LVHW070555100526
838202LV00012B/477